# BULLSEYE OR BULLSHIT

## CUT THROUGH THE MYTHS AND MAKE SMARTER FITNESS CHOICES

# RAJESH KUNDURI

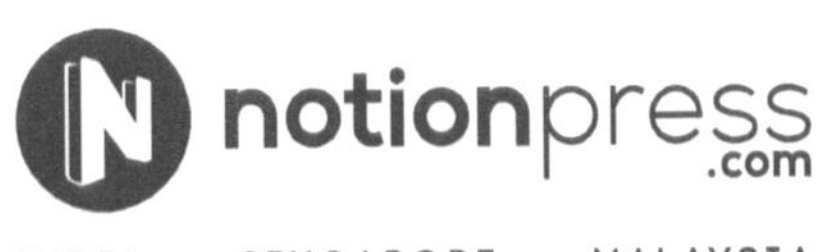

ISBN
Paperback  979-8-89556-811-8
Hardcase  979-8-89588-622-9

# Table of Contents

# Introduction

# Introduction: Bulls Eye or Bullshit?

In today's world, we are bombarded with endless information about fitness, health, and nutrition. It's like being in a huge, noisy market where everyone is shouting different advice. With so many voices, it's hard to know what really works and what's just a lot of hype. This book, "Bulls Eye or Bullshit?", is here to help you cut through the noise and get to the heart of what truly matters in your quest for better health and fitness.

## Why This Book?

You might be asking, "Why another fitness book?" The answer is simple: there's a lot of misleading information out there. Some of it sounds convincing but doesn't hold up when you dig deeper. Our goal is to provide clear, practical advice based on real science and proven methods. We want you to make informed decisions that actually work for you.

## What You'll Learn

This book covers a wide range of topics to help you understand and improve your fitness. Here's a sneak peek at what you can expect

1.  **The Basics of Fitness:** We'll start by exploring the fundamental principles of exercise and nutrition. You'll learn how your body responds to different types of workouts, what you should be eating to support your fitness goals, and how to set goals that are achievable and meaningful.

2.  **Personalizing Your Fitness Plan:** Fitness isn't one-size-fits-all. We'll guide you on how to tailor your workouts and diet to suit your unique needs. Whether you're a teenager, in your twenties, or well into your senior years, there's advice here for you. Your fitness plan should adapt to your age, lifestyle, and personal goals.

3.  **Separating Fact from Fiction in Nutrition:** Nutrition advice can be confusing. We'll debunk common myths and provide you with clear, science-backed information on what to eat. From understanding macronutrients like protein and carbs to knowing what supplements are worth your time, we've got you covered.

4.  **The Role of Mindset and Habits:** Achieving and maintaining fitness goals is as much about your mindset as it is about physical effort. We'll discuss how to build habits that stick and how to stay motivated even when you hit a rough patch.

5.  **Building a Support System:** Having the right support can make a huge difference. We'll talk

about how friends, family, and professional coaches can help you stay on track. Plus, we'll explore how to find and use online communities to keep yourself motivated and accountable.

6. **Embracing Technology:** Fitness technology is constantly evolving. We'll look at how apps and wearables can help you track your progress and improve your performance. Understanding how to use these tools effectively can give you an edge in reaching your fitness goals.

7. **Long-Term Fitness Success:** Fitness is a lifelong journey. We'll discuss strategies for maintaining your health and fitness over the long term, including how to adjust your routines as your life and goals change.

## Why It Matters

You might wonder why it's important to focus on getting accurate information and practical advice. Here's why:

1. **Avoiding Confusion:** With so many trends and fads, it's easy to get confused and overwhelmed. This book will help you cut through the clutter and focus on what really works.

2. **Making Informed Choices:** When you understand the science behind fitness and nutrition, you

can make better decisions about your health. This means you'll spend your time and effort on activities that genuinely benefit you.

3.  **Achieving Real Results:** Our goal is to help you achieve real, lasting results. By following the advice in this book, you'll be able to create a fitness plan that works for you and helps you reach your goals.

4.  **Enjoying the Process:** Fitness should be something you enjoy and look forward to. With the right knowledge and support, you can make your journey to better health a positive and rewarding experience.

## How to Use This Book

As you read through "Bulls Eye or Bullshit?", think of it as a practical guide rather than just theoretical advice. Each chapter is designed to give you actionable tips and insights that you can apply to your own fitness journey. Feel free to take notes, revisit sections, and adapt the advice to fit your personal needs and circumstances.

In summary, this book is here to help you navigate the often confusing world of fitness and nutrition. We aim to provide you with straightforward, practical advice that will help you make informed decisions and achieve your health and fitness goals. Welcome to **"Bulls Eye or Bullshit?"** — let's get started on the path to a healthier you!

# Exercise and Workouts

# Sequence of Exercise

Establishing an effective exercise routine requires attention to the order of exercises and the types of movements performed. Following a structured sequence helps maximize performance, minimize the risk of injury, and enhance overall results. Here's a comprehensive guide to the ideal sequence of exercises, along with examples.

## 1. Psychological Training

Before physical activity begins, it's beneficial to engage in **psychological training**. This involves techniques like visualization and concentration to mentally prepare for your workout. For example, visualize yourself successfully completing each exercise, which can boost confidence and performance.

## 2. Warm-Up

Next, initiate a **warm-up** session to prepare your body for the upcoming workout. This could include 5-10 minutes of light cardiovascular activity, such as jogging or cycling, to elevate your heart rate and increase blood flow to your muscles.

## 3. Dynamic Flexibility Training

After warming up, engage in **dynamic flexibility training**. This involves controlled movements that improve range of motion. For example, leg swings, arm circles, and torso twists are excellent dynamic stretches to enhance mobility.

## 4. Multiple-Joint Movements

Now, focus on **multiple-joint movements** that engage larger muscle groups. This stage is crucial for building strength and functional fitness.

- **Squats:** A fundamental exercise that targets the quadriceps, hamstrings, and glutes.

- **Bench Press:** Works primarily on the chest and triceps while also engaging the shoulders.

- **Dips:** A compound movement that targets the chest, shoulders, and triceps, enhancing upper body strength.

- **Overhead Press:** Strengthens the shoulders and upper back while also engaging the core.

## 5. Single-Joint Movements (Isolation)

Once multiple-joint movements are completed, transition to **single-joint movements**, which isolate specific muscles for focused strength development.

> **Larger Muscles:**

- **Chest/Back:** Exercises such as the chest fly (for the chest) or bent-over rows (for the back) specifically target these larger muscle groups.

> **Smaller Muscles:**

- **Biceps/Triceps/Deltoids:** Incorporate exercises like bicep curls for the biceps, tricep extensions for the triceps, and lateral raises for the deltoids to strengthen these smaller muscle groups.

## 6. Flexibility Training

Following the strength exercises, engage in **flexibility training**. This includes static stretching, which helps improve flexibility and aids in recovery. Focus on stretches that target the muscles worked during your session, such as holding a quad stretch or a hamstring stretch.

## 7. Cooldown

A proper **cooldown** is essential to help your body gradually return to its resting state. This can involve 5-10 minutes of light activity, followed by gentle stretches to relax the muscles.

## 8. Application of Appropriate Therapy

Finally, consider the **application of appropriate therapy** if needed. This could include methods such as ice treatment to reduce inflammation, TENS (Transcutaneous Electrical Nerve Stimulation) for pain relief, or foam rolling to alleviate muscle tightness.

# Zumba: Dance or Exercise?

When traditional dance forms like Kuchipudi, Kathakali, and Bharatanatyam aren't recognized as exercises despite their physically demanding routines, it raises the question: Why is Zumba glorified as a fitness solution? Unlike these traditional dances, Zumba has been aggressively marketed as a fun and effective way to lose weight and stay fit, but the reality is more nuanced.

## Accessibility and Cost-Effectiveness

One of the reasons Zumba gained rapid popularity is its accessibility and low setup cost. While setting up a high-end gym involves significant investment—costing crores in equipment, maintenance, and space requirements—a Zumba center only needs an empty space and a set of audio speakers. A single trainer can lead sessions for tens or even hundreds of participants, making it a cost-effective alternative to traditional gyms. This simplicity and lower cost structure contribute to its widespread appeal, especially for those looking for a more affordable and sociable way to stay active.

## Does Zumba Have a Place in Fitness?

Zumba can indeed be part of a fitness routine, especially if you love dancing and find joy in it. If dancing elevates your mood, helps you unwind, and makes you look forward to exercising, then Zumba can be a great fit for you. It provides a cardio workout that can improve endurance and offers a fun way to socialize with others who share your passion.

However, it's important to recognize that while Zumba is enjoyable, it should not be viewed as a complete solution for achieving long-term fitness goals. Zumba primarily focuses on cardiovascular health but lacks the muscle-building benefits that strength training provides. To truly maximize your fitness results, the better strategy is to combine Zumba with other forms of exercise, such as weight training or high-intensity interval training (HIIT). This approach brings the best of both worlds: the fun and sociability of Zumba, along with the strength and metabolic boosts from more intensive exercises.

## A Balanced Fitness Approach

Ultimately, the key to achieving and maintaining fitness lies in a balanced approach. Enjoy Zumba for what it offers—an engaging, mood-boosting dance workout—but also incorporate other activities that build strength, flexibility, and overall health. By combining Zumba with weight training or other structured exercise routines, you can create a comprehensive fitness plan that supports your goals, keeps you motivated, and most importantly, makes your journey enjoyable.

# Yoga: Meditation or Modern Fitness Solution?

Yoga has its roots deeply embedded in ancient Indian traditions, originally practiced as a form of meditation and spiritual discipline rather than a modern exercise regimen. With the evolution of science and fitness, questions arise about the relevance of traditional practices like Yoga. Just as you wouldn't send your child to a Sanskrit-only school today, clinging to outdated practices without understanding their modern context may not be the best approach.

## The Evolution of Yoga

Traditional Yoga, as taught by ancient sages like Vishwamitra to Rama, was often conducted in a one-on-one setting, tailored to individual needs. It was never about group classes in studios or wearing trendy yoga pants; it was about discipline, mental focus, and spiritual growth. Today, Yoga has been significantly modified to fit contemporary fitness culture, often being marketed as a one-size-fits-all solution for flexibility, stress relief, and even weight loss.

# The Misconception of Yoga for Flexibility and Weight Loss

Many turn to Yoga in hopes of regaining lost flexibility or for weight loss, believing it's the ultimate solution. However, Yoga is generally a low-intensity activity that might not be as effective for these goals when compared to other forms of exercise like strength training or HIIT (High-Intensity Interval Training). Research shows that Yoga can improve flexibility and mobility to some extent, but these gains are often limited compared to more targeted flexibility or mobility training routines.

For example, a study published in the "Journal of Physical Therapy Science" found that while Yoga can improve flexibility, other exercises specifically designed for mobility training offer more significant results over the same period . Additionally, Yoga's gentle movements may not raise the heart rate sufficiently to contribute significantly to weight loss compared to more vigorous activities.

## Stress Reduction: The Reality Check

Yoga is often praised for its stress-relieving benefits, but in a world where stressors like delayed paychecks, traffic jams, or even seeing an accident on the road are common, the efficacy of Yoga as a primary stress management tool can be limited. The physiological impact of Yoga might not always match the immediate demands of these real-world stressors.

## A Sustainable Approach

If you enjoy Yoga and find solace in its practices, it can undoubtedly be part of a sustainable lifestyle. It offers mental relaxation, improves mindfulness, and can complement other fitness routines. However, if your primary goal is weight loss or intensive flexibility gains, incorporating Yoga with other exercises that specifically target these needs would be a more effective strategy.

## Conclusion: Yoga in Modern Fitness

While Yoga has a place in modern fitness, especially for those who enjoy its meditative aspects, it shouldn't be viewed as a standalone solution for all fitness goals. Recognizing its limitations and integrating it with other forms of exercise will provide a more balanced and effective approach to health and wellness.

## References

Thomas, E., et al. (2017). "The effects of yoga on flexibility: A systematic review." *Journal of Strength and Conditioning Research*, 31(12), 3338-3345.

Advanced Human Performance. (n.d.). "The Truth About Yoga: Flexibility & Mobility Training." Retrieved from Advanced Human Performance

# Karate, Kung Fu, and Kickboxing: The Reality Behind the Moves

Martial arts like Karate, Kung Fu, and Kickboxing have long been celebrated for their disciplined approach to self-defense, fitness, and even weight loss. However, it's essential to differentiate the choreographed moves seen in movies from real-life scenarios. In films, fights are meticulously planned to look impressive and dramatic, but real confrontations are unpredictable, and the effectiveness of traditional martial arts techniques in actual self-defense situations can be questionable.

## The Limitations of Traditional Techniques

Training in martial arts often involves repetitive practice of blocks, punches, and kicks, following structured patterns like X-blocks or Y-blocks. However, these techniques may not prepare you for real-world threats, such as a stone being thrown or, more critically, a bullet fired from a rifle. The reality is that martial arts were historically developed for specific contexts—like protecting temples or engaging in hand-to-hand combat centuries ago. While they may have been relevant then, these practices do not necessarily translate effectively to modern-day self-defense needs where threats can involve firearms or unexpected violence.

## Outdated Practices for Modern Challenges

Martial arts like Kung Fu were originally developed to protect temples and for personal defense in times when hand-to-hand combat was more common. However, the nature of self-defense has evolved significantly. Relying solely on traditional martial arts for self-protection today may not be the most practical approach, especially when faced with threats beyond fist-to-fist combat. The structured and ceremonial moves practiced over years may not provide the spontaneous, adaptive responses needed in real danger.

## Martial Arts and Weight Loss: A Misguided Path?

Many people also turn to martial arts like Karate and Kickboxing for weight loss, lured by the high-energy workouts and the allure of learning self-defense. However, while these activities can be intense and burn calories, they might not be the most efficient path to weight loss compared to more targeted fitness regimens. High-intensity interval training (HIIT), strength training, and cardio exercises are often more effective for fat loss and muscle building. The martial arts training environment can sometimes create a false sense of security, both in terms of physical self-defense and fitness results.

## A Balanced Perspective on Martial Arts

If you enjoy practicing Karate, Kung Fu, or Kickboxing, they can still be valuable as part of your fitness routine, offering benefits like improved discipline, coordination, and physical conditioning. However, it's important to understand their limitations and not view them as the ultimate solution for self-defense or weight loss. Combining martial arts with other fitness and self-defense methods, such as situational awareness training or mixed martial arts (MMA), can provide a more comprehensive approach to personal safety and health.

## Conclusion: Martial Arts in Modern Fitness and Self-Defense

Martial arts have their place as cultural practices and personal hobbies, but it's crucial to recognize that they are not a one-size-fits-all solution for modern self-defense or fitness. Adapting to current challenges with a broader, more practical approach can ensure that your time and effort are effectively aligned with your personal goals.

# Walking: More Than Just Putting One Foot in Front of the Other?

Walking is often promoted as the simplest form of exercise—just put on a pair of sneakers and hit the pavement. But let's take a step back and consider the broader picture. Our grandparents never needed a specific time or gear to walk for exercise; they simply incorporated it into their daily lives, whether through chores, farming, or commuting. Nature equipped fish with fins and birds with wings, yet they don't fly around for exactly 30 minutes each day in the name of exercise. The human body, similarly, was designed to move in varied ways, not just to walk as a prescribed form of fitness.

## The Hidden Risks of Walking

Walking is accessible to nearly everyone with two legs, but it's not without its risks, especially when not done mindfully. For instance, overweight individuals may experience an additional 30% increase in knee joint pressure with each step, potentially leading to conditions like knee osteoarthritis over time. While walking seems like a no-brainer because "anyone can do it," the impact on joints, especially when carrying extra weight, should not be underestimated.

# Walking vs. Other Activities: The Confidence Factor

Walking inherently instills confidence because it's something we all learn from a young age. Unlike swimming, which requires specific skills, or using gym equipment, which often necessitates guidance, walking feels natural and straightforward. There's no need for special training or overcoming the fear of doing something new. But does this ease mean it's the best form of exercise for everyone? Not necessarily.

# The Treadmill: From Punishment to Fitness Tool

Interestingly, the treadmill, now a staple in modern gyms, has a darker history. Originally known as the "treadwheel," it was used as a punishment device in 19th-century prisons, forcing inmates to walk for hours as a form of hard labor. It's ironic that a device once used to instill discipline and toil has now been repurposed as a symbol of fitness and health.

# A Balanced View on Walking

While walking is undoubtedly a beneficial activity, especially for those who enjoy it and find it sustainable, it's important to recognize that it might not be sufficient on its own for comprehensive fitness. Like any other form of exercise, it has its place but should ideally be combined with other activities that challenge the body in different ways, such as strength training, swimming, or cycling, for a more rounded approach to health.

## Conclusion: Walking as Part of a Broader Fitness Strategy

Walking is easy, accessible, and familiar—qualities that make it appealing to many. However, it's essential to view it as one piece of a larger fitness puzzle rather than the entire solution. Integrating walking with a variety of other exercises that cater to individual goals and physical needs will ultimately lead to better health outcomes and a more enjoyable fitness journey.

# Cycling: Commute or Exercise?

Cycling was originally invented as a practical solution for commuting long distances, not as a means for fitness enthusiasts to pedal aimlessly for the sake of weight loss. Ask yourself this: Did your grandfather hop on a cycle just to burn calories, or did he use it for the purpose it was intended—transportation? When choosing exercises, it's essential to apply relevance and context.

## The Reality of Long-Distance Cycling

If you observe long-distance cyclists, marathon runners, or endurance athletes, you'll notice a common trend: they are often lean to the point of being "skinny to the bone." This is a direct result of the type of training they engage in. Long-distance cycling and similar endurance activities focus on cardiovascular fitness, burning calories but doing little to build muscle mass. While great for stamina, it can leave out key aspects of a balanced fitness routine, such as strength building.

## The Key: Combining Strength and Endurance

To maximize the benefits of cycling, it's wise to pair it with weight training. While cycling can build endurance and cardiovascular health, weight training adds strength, helping you build muscle and improve overall fitness. This combination allows you to harness the best of both worlds—endurance from cycling and strength from resistance training.

## Conclusion: Cycle with Purpose

Cycling has its place, whether for commuting or cardio workouts, but as with any form of exercise, it's crucial to contextualize it within your broader fitness goals. By combining cycling with strength training, you create a more comprehensive fitness routine that builds both endurance and strength, leading to better long-term health outcomes.

# Fitness Science and Concepts

# What is Fitness?

Looking fit and being fit are two completely different worlds. Society often equates fitness with appearance, but reality paints a different picture. You might see someone who looks lean and slim but has dangerously high levels of visceral fat—fat that wraps around internal organs and contributes to severe health issues. On the other hand, someone with a muscular, bulky build could have low testosterone or other hormone imbalances that affect their overall health. Clearly, fitness isn't just about how your body looks on the outside; it's about how it functions on the inside.

Athletes, for example, come in all shapes and sizes. A 140 kg bodybuilder is celebrated for their muscle mass and strength, while a 200 kg sumo wrestler is recognized for agility and technique. Why are they awarded and rewarded despite their vastly different physiques? Because fitness is about what your body can *do*, not just how it looks. The point is, fitness is multidimensional—it's not limited to a specific body type or appearance.

## The Real Definition of Fitness

Fitness should be about more than losing a few kilograms for a fleeting Instagram post. It should translate into real-life abilities and functionality. Can you push a car when it's stuck on a slope? Can you climb 10 flights of stairs when the elevator isn't working? Do you have the stamina to play with your kids, the strength to carry your groceries, or the mobility to get in and out of a chair without discomfort? These are the true measures of fitness that directly impact your quality of life.

It's easy to get caught up in the pursuit of aesthetics— chasing after six-pack abs or the perfect beach body. But real fitness goes beyond that. True fitness is having the strength, endurance, and flexibility to navigate life's physical challenges with ease. It's being able to move, sit, lift, and perform day-to-day activities without pain or strain. These abilities are a better indicator of your overall health than any number on a scale or likes on a social media post.

## Fitness for the Long Run: Functional Health

Fitness isn't just about building muscles or burning fat; it's about building a body that works well for your lifestyle. Having strong bones, maintaining an optimal balance of muscle mass and fat, and developing the mobility to move freely without restriction—these are the pillars of long-term health and fitness. Your body should be resilient and adaptable, ready to take on both everyday tasks and unexpected physical demands.

Think about what you need in your life. If you're a parent, fitness means being able to lift your child without hurting your back. If you're aging, fitness might mean maintaining bone density and muscle mass to reduce the risk of injury or falls. Your fitness goals should align with your real-world needs, not some idealized version of fitness that's limited to how your body looks.

## Conclusion: Fitness is Functionality

In the end, fitness is about functionality. It's not about fitting into a certain aesthetic mold, but about developing a body that serves you in your daily life. Whether it's lifting, moving, pushing, or pulling, fitness should help you handle the challenges that life throws at you. Real fitness is about being physically capable and resilient—ready for whatever life has in store.

# Is Bodybuilding the Only Way?

Absolutely not. When I say strength training is crucial, I'm not suggesting you start sculpting your body like an idol, meticulously naming every day "Leg Day," "Biceps Day," or "Chest Day." What I am saying is that strength—genuine, functional strength—has always been at the core of human survival and health. Think about it: our ancestors didn't hit the gym, but they engaged in grueling labor, built wonders like the Taj Mahal, fortresses, and temples by hauling stones and bricks on their shoulders. They drew water from wells, using their arms and latissimus dorsi muscles without a second thought. How healthy were they?

If you look back, the rates of diseases and mortality were at historic lows compared to modern sedentary lifestyles. There's a reason why they thrived.

## Strength is the Foundation of Longevity

All I'm advocating for is to **be strong** and **become stronger**—because true strength offers a unique functionality. It's not just about vanity muscles or flexing in the mirror. Strength training through lifting heavy weights changes your body composition, boosts your hormonal balance, and keeps you young, fit, and active. Strength ensures that your body stays robust, resilient, and efficient. **You won't age the same way when you have a strong, functional body.**

When you engage in strength training, particularly compound movements like deadlifts, squats, and bench presses, you challenge multiple muscle groups at once. Progressive overload—gradually increasing the weight you lift—helps build endurance, mobility, flexibility, and a well-rounded physique. The time you invest in weight training offers the best return on investment (ROI) when it comes to exercise. It is not about focusing on one muscle at a time, but about building your entire body's capacity to handle life's physical demands.

## The Metabolic Boost of Strength Training

Unlike aerobics or other forms of exercise that give you a short-term calorie burn, **strength training turns you into a calorie-burning machine** even when you're doing nothing. After a weightlifting session, your metabolism remains elevated for the next 36 to 48 hours, meaning your body burns more calories while you sleep, sit, or simply relax. This is the magic of resistance training—it doesn't just build muscles; it enhances your body's ability to burn fat and sustain a healthy metabolic rate.

## Conclusion: Strength Training for Life

So, no, bodybuilding isn't the only way, but building strength should be a priority. Weight training offers more than just muscle; it offers longevity, health, and functionality. You can achieve strength, endurance, mobility, flexibility, and a well-rounded fitness level just by having a well-structured plan and lifting weights. It's the most effective way to ensure your body stays in optimal condition, no matter your age or goals.

# How to Make Your Workout Plan in the Gym

Creating an effective workout plan involves more than just selecting random exercises. To maximize your performance and results, you need to follow a structured approach that ensures you target all necessary aspects of fitness, from strength to flexibility. Below are essential steps and a logical order to follow when planning your workout in the gym.

## 1. Psychological Training

Start with **mental preparation**—visualization and concentration exercises. This step helps you get into the right mindset for the workout, boosting motivation and focus. Mental training can include visualizing your movements, thinking about your goals, or practicing mindfulness to increase focus and lower stress levels.

## 2. Warm-up

Always begin with a proper warm-up to prepare your muscles, joints, and cardiovascular system for more intense activity. A 5–10 minute session of light cardio (e.g., brisk walking, cycling, or skipping) will raise your heart rate and body temperature, increasing blood flow to the muscles and reducing the risk of injury.

## 3. Dynamic Flexibility Training

Before jumping into weightlifting or explosive movements, do **dynamic stretching** to loosen up your muscles and improve your range of motion. Exercises like leg swings, arm circles, or walking lunges get your body ready for action while preventing stiffness and injury.

## 4. Explosive Training (if applicable)

If your goal includes power or athletic performance, include **explosive training** early in your session. This could involve CAT (Compensatory Acceleration Training), Olympic lifts, plyometrics (like box jumps), or sprint drills. These exercises require maximum effort and speed, so they should be performed when you're fresh.

## 5. Multiple-Joint Movements (Compound Exercises)

Next, focus on **compound movements**, which involve multiple muscle groups and joints. These are the foundation of any strength training program because they stimulate the most muscle growth and strength.

- **Squats** (Target: legs, core)

- **Deadlifts** (Target: back, legs, core)

- **Bench Press** (Target: chest, shoulders, triceps)

- **Dips, Overhead Press** (Target: upper body)

Start with heavier weights and lower repetitions (4–8 reps) to focus on building strength and muscle.

## 6. Single-Joint Movements (Isolation Exercises)

After compound lifts, move on to **isolation exercises** that target specific muscles. This phase allows you to focus on muscles that may not have been fully worked during the compound lifts. Perform these exercises with a moderate number of repetitions (8–12 reps) for hypertrophy (muscle growth).

- **Larger muscles**: Quads, hamstrings, chest, back.

- **Smaller muscles**: Biceps, triceps, calves, shoulders.

## 7. Flexibility Training (Static Stretching)

After all the heavy lifting and muscle fatigue, cool down with **static stretching**. This helps improve flexibility, prevent injury, and aids in muscle recovery. Use techniques like SFMR (Stretching, Fascial Mobility, Release) to focus on improving joint mobility.

## 8. Cooldown

Finish your workout with a **cooldown** to gradually bring your heart rate down. This can be a few minutes of light cardio and more stretching, which helps flush out lactic acid and promotes faster recovery.

## 9. Application of Therapy (if needed)

If you've had an intense session or are feeling sore, use recovery techniques such as:

- **Ice treatment**: Helps reduce inflammation.

- **TENS (Transcutaneous Electrical Nerve Stimulation)**: Can help alleviate pain or muscle soreness post-workout.

- **Massage**: Promotes blood flow and muscle recovery.

# Machines vs. Free Weights

When it comes to choosing between machines and free weights, one major difference stands out: **machines are designed to fit everyone into a specific, predetermined movement pattern**. Whether you're tall, short, lean, or heavy, the machine's structure dictates how you perform the exercise, often without considering the uniqueness of your body. While machines can be easy and convenient to use, they come with limitations that free weights can overcome.

Machines are appealing for beginners because they offer **guidance and stability**. They help isolate specific muscles and reduce the risk of poor form, making them ideal for those unfamiliar with strength training. However, this simplicity comes with a downside. Machines often force your body into a movement path that may not be natural for your joints. Over time, this lack of joint flexibility can lead to strain or injury, as the machine doesn't adapt to your body – you have to adapt to the machine.

On the other hand, **free weights offer versatility and functionality**. With free weights like dumbbells, barbells, and kettlebells, you can move in a more natural range of motion, making the exercise more joint-friendly. Your body is free to follow its own path, engaging stabilizer muscles to support and balance the movement. This not only reduces injury risk but also builds strength that translates better to real-world activities, where you need to control your body in unpredictable environments.

Additionally, **free weights provide greater functional benefits**. While machines isolate muscles, free weights involve multiple muscle groups, promoting better coordination, balance, and core strength. Whether you're pushing, pulling, or lifting, you're working your entire body in harmony, something machines can't replicate.

While machines have their place in rehab or specific muscle isolation, relying solely on them can limit your overall fitness potential. **Free weights offer a broader range of motion, better joint protection, and more functional strength**, making them a superior choice for long-term strength gains.

# Swimming: The Ultimate Joint-Friendly Exercise

Swimming is one of the most effective and joint-friendly exercises, offering a unique **3D support to your body**. Unlike land-based activities, swimming provides a low-impact environment where water cushions your movements, significantly reducing the stress placed on your joints. This makes it an ideal option, especially for individuals recovering from injuries or those with joint conditions like arthritis.

Water provides **natural resistance**, but without the harsh contact forces that come with running or jumping on hard surfaces. When you swim, your body is supported in all directions, minimizing the risk of impact-related injuries while still providing a great workout. This buoyancy not only allows you to move more freely but also encourages a full range of motion, enhancing joint flexibility and mobility. The resistance of water helps strengthen muscles without placing undue strain on your skeletal system, making swimming perfect for injury rehabilitation.

In addition to being gentle on the joints, swimming is a **primitive yet highly effective sport** that has been practiced for centuries. It's one of the few forms of exercise that works your entire body—arms, legs, core, and cardiovascular system—all at once. This full-body engagement, combined with the joint support water provides, makes swimming an excellent choice for maintaining or improving fitness, even when high-impact exercises aren't an option.

Moreover, the **reduced friction in water** compared to the ground enables smooth, continuous movements, further minimizing the wear and tear on your body. Whether you're recovering from an injury, looking to protect your joints, or simply seeking a versatile workout, swimming is a **gentle but powerful option** that delivers both cardiovascular and muscular benefits with minimal risk to your joints.

# Law of Thermodynamics: The Basics of Weight Management

The **Law of Thermodynamics** offers a clear-cut view on weight management that hinges on a straightforward principle: **calories in versus calories out**. This law states that:

> **Consuming more calories than you expend** leads to weight gain.

> **Consuming the same number of calories as you burn** will keep your weight stable.

> **Consuming fewer calories than you burn** results in weight loss.

This principle remains true regardless of diet trends or exercise fads. You might experiment with fasting, eat minimally, or indulge in a 300-calorie cake, and you might not witness immediate changes in your body. This delay can often lead people to overlook the importance of consistent, long-term habits in achieving and maintaining good health.

Health and fitness are not defined by the effects of a single meal or a short-term regimen. Just as regularly consuming alcohol can lead to alcoholism over time, or daily smoking can severely damage your lungs, your overall health is the result of your cumulative choices and behaviors. One healthy carrot or one indulgent slice of cake will not significantly impact your body; it's the consistent pattern of your habits that determines your health and fitness outcomes.

**Repetition and consistency** are crucial. A single bicep curl or one gym session won't make you fit, just as one day of skipping exercise won't cause immediate decline. Instead, it's the accumulation of efforts over time that leads to noticeable changes. Committing to regular exercise and maintaining a balanced diet over several months will result in a significant transformation.

Ultimately, your body is a reflection of your daily habits. Success in health and fitness comes from the steady, consistent application of positive habits rather than sporadic, extreme efforts or indulgences. Focus on building and maintaining these habits, and you'll see long-term benefits that reflect in your physical health and overall well-being.

# How Much to Eat: Practical Guidelines for Balanced Nutrition

Understanding how much to eat is crucial for maintaining a healthy diet and managing body weight. This concept can be illustrated through a straightforward, practical guide that focuses on intuitive portions rather than complex calorie counting.

| Visual Cues for Portion Sizes: |
| --- |
| **Protein:** |
| **Size:** A portion should be the size of your palm.<br><br>**Example:** Think of a beggar holding out their hand, asking for food. The space between their fingers gives a clear picture of how much protein you should aim for—about the same size as your own palm. This includes sources such as chicken, fish, tofu, or legumes. Protein is essential for muscle repair and growth, making it a vital component of your meals. |
| Vegetables: |
| **Size:** A portion should be the size of your fist.<br><br>**Example:** Fill half your plate with a variety of colorful vegetables like spinach, bell peppers, broccoli, or carrots. Vegetables are packed with vitamins, minerals, and fiber, which are crucial for overall health. |

| **Fat:** |
|---|
| **Size:** Keep this portion the size of your thumb.<br><br>**Example:** Healthy fats come from sources like olive oil, nuts, seeds, or avocado. Fats are important for hormone production and nutrient absorption, but it's key to consume them in moderation. |
| **Carbohydrates:** |
| **Size:** A portion should be the size of your cupped hand.<br><br>**Example:** Choose whole grains such as brown rice, quinoa, or whole-grain bread. Carbohydrates are your body's primary energy source, especially important for fueling workouts. |

## Incorporating Intuitive Eating Concepts:

This approach to portion control draws inspiration from traditional dietary practices and emphasizes common sense. The goal is to create balanced meals that are nutrient-dense while being satisfying.

## Practical Application:

➤ **Visualize Your Plate:** When preparing meals, use these guidelines to help fill your plate with appropriate portions. Picture each section of your plate representing the visual cues discussed—this method helps manage your intake without needing precise measurements or calorie counting.

> **Listen to Your Body:** Eat until you're satisfied, not overly full. These portion sizes are guidelines, and individual needs may vary based on activity level, metabolic rate, and health goals.

> **Mindful Eating:** Pay attention to the quality of the food you consume. Opt for whole, unprocessed foods whenever possible, and make sure to incorporate a variety of nutrients in each meal.

By using these simple visual cues, you can make healthier eating choices that align with your nutritional needs while avoiding the complexities of detailed dietary tracking. This balanced approach supports overall health and well-being, making it easier to maintain a nutritious diet.

# RDA vs. PDI: Understanding Individual Nutritional Needs

The Recommended Dietary Allowances (RDA) and Personal Dietary Intake (PDI) guidelines provide general benchmarks for nutrition, but they don't account for the full spectrum of individual needs and performance requirements. Let's explore why these recommendations might fall short for some people and how they can be tailored to fit individual needs.

1. **Standard Work Hours and Performance:** The traditional 8-5 workday is a standard designed to fit a broad range of jobs and industries. However, cognitive and physical performance can vary significantly among individuals. Some people can complete tasks more efficiently and with greater creativity, potentially achieving faster results than others. The idea that everyone should adhere to the same work hours overlooks the fact that productivity and efficiency are influenced by personal work habits, job roles, and cognitive strengths. Customizing work schedules and allowing flexibility can lead to better performance and well-being.

2. **Hydration Recommendations:** The general guideline to drink 3-4 liters of water daily is

based on average needs, but individual hydration requirements can vary. Factors such as body size, physical activity, climate, and health conditions influence water needs. Athletes, for instance, may require more water due to increased sweat loss, while sedentary individuals in cooler climates might need less. Personal hydration should be adjusted based on activity levels and environmental conditions, rather than a one-size-fits-all recommendation.

3. **Protein Intake:** The standard recommendation of 0.86 grams of protein per kilogram of body weight is designed for the average adult. However, this doesn't account for variations in physical activity or body composition. A construction worker or an athlete who engages in intense physical activity requires more protein to support muscle repair, recovery, and overall performance. Tailoring protein intake to match physical demands helps optimize performance and recovery, ensuring that dietary needs are met based on individual activity levels and goals.

4. **Specialized Nutritional Needs:** High-performance individuals, such as marathon runners, professional athletes like Virat Kohli, or strongmen lifting heavy weights, have unique nutritional requirements. Their bodies demand

more energy, salt, minerals, and other nutrients to sustain their performance and recovery. For example, a marathon runner's needs will differ significantly from someone with a sedentary lifestyle, requiring more carbohydrates for energy and electrolytes to replace losses from prolonged exertion.

5. **Food as Fuel:** Recognizing that food is fuel for your body, it's important to adjust your intake based on performance and activity levels. Instead of adhering strictly to general guidelines, personalize your diet to support your specific needs and goals. This might involve increasing your intake of certain nutrients or adjusting macronutrient ratios to better suit your physical demands.

In conclusion, while RDAs provide valuable general guidelines, they are not always sufficient for meeting individual needs. Personalizing your diet and lifestyle based on your unique performance requirements, activity levels, and health goals will help you achieve optimal health and performance. Embrace the flexibility to break away from standard recommendations and tailor your nutrition to fit your individual needs for better overall results.

# Food Pyramid: Embracing Sustainable Practices and Cultural Diversity

The concept of the Food Pyramid has long been used to guide nutritional choices, often emphasizing a balanced diet rich in fruits, vegetables, whole grains, and lean proteins. However, this model can sometimes oversimplify the diverse dietary practices that vary across cultures and regions. Let's delve into how sustainable practices and cultural traditions shape our food choices and why these should be considered alongside general dietary guidelines.

1. **Cultural Dietary Practices:** Different regions around the world have unique culinary traditions that are closely linked to their local environments and cultural heritage. For instance, coastal countries typically include fish as a staple in their diets due to its availability and nutritional benefits. In Italy, pizza reflects local ingredients and traditional cooking methods, while South Indians might favor idly, sambar, and rice, staples that have been integral to their diet for generations.

2. **Historical Eating Patterns:** Historical eating patterns often provide insight into sustainable and healthful food choices. For example, many

traditional diets were based on locally available ingredients and seasonal produce. Your grandmother's diet might have included rice, chikki, and sweets made for religious offerings and enjoyed as prasad. These foods were not only culturally significant but also suited to the local environment and available resources.

3. **Sustainability and Local Food Systems:** Embracing local food systems and sustainable practices is essential for both environmental health and personal well-being. Foods like fish in coastal areas or grains in more arid regions are often chosen because they are sustainable and well-suited to the local ecosystem. Adapting the Food Pyramid to include local and culturally significant foods can help support regional agriculture and reduce environmental impact.

4. **Modern Adaptations:** While the traditional Food Pyramid provides a basic framework for nutrition, integrating local food practices and personal preferences can enhance its relevance. For instance, incorporating traditional dishes that align with modern nutritional understanding can create a more culturally resonant and sustainable diet. Instead of rigidly following the pyramid, consider how your dietary choices can reflect both

your cultural heritage and current nutritional needs.

5. **Balancing Tradition and Modernity:** Balancing traditional dietary practices with modern nutritional science can offer a more comprehensive approach to health. While the Food Pyramid provides a general guideline, respecting cultural traditions and local food systems can lead to more satisfying and sustainable eating habits. This approach not only honors historical and cultural contexts but also supports a diverse and balanced diet.

In summary, while the Food Pyramid offers useful guidance for a balanced diet, it is important to integrate sustainable practices and respect cultural food traditions. Embracing local foods and historical dietary patterns can contribute to a healthier and more environmentally friendly way of eating. By combining traditional wisdom with contemporary nutritional knowledge, we can create a more holistic approach to diet and well-being.

# Evolution and Distribution of Food: From Sacred to Vilified

Throughout history, food has held a deep significance across cultures, often intertwined with religious and cultural practices. Fruits and other natural foods have been celebrated and revered for their health benefits and symbolic meanings. However, in modern times, some foods, especially fruits, have faced unwarranted criticism, particularly regarding their sugar content. Let's explore the evolution of food perceptions and the misinterpretation of natural sugars.

1. **Historical and Religious Significance:** Foods have always played a crucial role in religious and cultural contexts. For instance, in the Bible, apples are often depicted as symbols of knowledge and temptation. The Quran mentions dates and figs as revered fruits, reflecting their historical importance in various cultures. Such references underscore the longstanding recognition of these foods as valuable and beneficial.

2. **Cultural Practices:** Across cultures, fruits have been used in rituals and offerings. For example, bananas are offered with agarbatti (incense) in many Hindu ceremonies, symbolizing purity and

prosperity. These practices highlight the respect and reverence historically afforded to fruits, recognizing them as integral to cultural and spiritual practices.

3. **Misconceptions about Natural Sugars:** In recent times, the narrative around sugar has become increasingly negative, with fruits sometimes being unjustly labeled as harmful due to their natural sugar content. This perspective often overlooks the fact that fruit sugars are naturally occurring and come with a host of beneficial nutrients like fiber, vitamins, and antioxidants. Comparing the sugar in fruits to refined sugars or processed foods is akin to comparing water in a swimming pool to water in a drinking glass—different contexts, different effects.

4. **The Role of Natural Sugars:** The sugar found in fruits is not the same as the added sugars found in processed foods. Fruit sugars are accompanied by fiber, which helps regulate blood sugar levels and provides a slower, more sustained release of energy. Additionally, fruits contain essential nutrients that contribute to overall health. The health benefits of consuming whole fruits far outweigh the potential concerns about their natural sugar content.

5. **Evolving Perceptions:** The shift in perceptions about fruits and their sugars often stems from

broader dietary trends and misconceptions. It is important to differentiate between natural and added sugars and to understand the context in which these sugars are consumed. Fruits, with their rich nutrient profiles, remain a crucial part of a balanced diet and should not be vilified based on misguided or oversimplified nutritional advice.

6. **Balancing Nutritional Understanding:** While it's essential to be mindful of overall sugar intake, it's equally important to recognize the value of natural foods in a balanced diet. Embracing a nuanced understanding of nutrition, which respects both historical significance and modern science, can lead to more informed dietary choices.

In summary, the evolution of food perceptions—from sacred and revered to criticized—reflects broader changes in dietary trends and misunderstandings about natural sugars. Fruits, with their rich cultural heritage and nutritional benefits, should be appreciated for their role in a healthy diet rather than unfairly criticized. Understanding the difference between natural and processed sugars helps maintain a balanced perspective on nutrition and respects the historical and cultural importance of these foods.

## Foods with Labels: A Double-Edged Sword

In today's market, the proliferation of food labels can be both confusing and misleading. From colorful packaging to buzzwords like "low-fat," "sugar-free," and "diabetes-friendly," labels are designed to catch our eye and influence our purchasing decisions. However, the healthiest foods don't come with labels, and understanding this distinction is crucial for making informed dietary choices. Here's a deeper look into why foods with labels might not always be as healthy as they seem and how to navigate this landscape effectively.

1. **The Reality of Unlabeled Foods:** The most nutritious foods are often those that don't come with flashy labels. Think of fresh fruits, vegetables, nuts, and grains—these whole foods are inherently healthy and don't need marketing gimmicks to prove their worth. You won't see celebrities endorsing "fresh tomatoes" or "organic carrots" with health claims because their benefits are well-established and universally acknowledged.

2. **The Marketing Strategy:** The colorful labels and health claims on packaged foods are designed to grab attention and create a perception of healthiness. Phrases like "high in protein," "baked, not fried," or "no added sugar" can be misleading. While these attributes might seem beneficial,

they don't always translate to overall health. For instance, "low-fat" snacks might be high in sugars or artificial additives, and "sugar-free" products might contain other unhealthy ingredients.

3. **The Truth Behind the Labels:** Labels often serve more as marketing tools than as indicators of true health benefits. For example, "diabetes-friendly biscuits" might be lower in sugar, but they could still contain refined flours and unhealthy fats. The packaging might boast about being "high in protein," but if it's processed and loaded with additives, it's far from a wholesome choice.

4. **The Appeal of Earthy Colors:** Many unhealthy foods are packaged in earthy tones and green colors to give a natural, healthy impression. This strategy can mislead consumers into thinking that the product is healthier than it actually is. The marketing of these foods often plays on the visual appeal rather than the actual nutritional value.

5. **Choosing Fresh Produce:** To avoid the pitfalls of misleading labels, consider shopping at local markets or "mandis" where you can find fresh, unprocessed produce. These foods are not only more nutrient-dense but also free from the marketing gimmicks that often accompany packaged goods. Fresh fruits, vegetables, and whole grains are straightforward in their health

benefits, providing essential nutrients without the need for labels.

6.  **The Bottom Line:** While labels can provide some useful information, they should not be the sole factor in determining the healthfulness of a food. It's essential to look beyond the marketing claims and focus on whole, unprocessed foods that offer genuine nutritional benefits. By shopping for fresh produce and being critical of the labels on packaged foods, you can make better choices that align with your health goals.

In conclusion, the healthiest foods are often those without labels, and understanding the motives behind food packaging can help you make more informed dietary decisions. Prioritize fresh, unprocessed produce and approach labeled products with a discerning eye to ensure that your diet supports your overall well-being.

# Eating Healthy Isn't the Goal: Tailoring Your Diet to Your Goals

Eating healthy is often touted as the ultimate goal in nutrition, but this approach overlooks a crucial aspect: aligning your diet with your specific health and fitness goals. It's not just about what's on your plate, but when and how it fits into your overall plan. Here's why focusing solely on healthy foods might not be enough, and how you can better tailor your diet to achieve your personal objectives.

1. **The Misconception of a "Healthy" Plate:** Picture a plate with two eggs, a glass of milk, a serving of dry fruits, two rotis with curry, and a banana. On the surface, this might seem like a balanced and nutritious meal. However, when you add up the calories, it becomes clear that this plate could contribute to an excess of daily caloric intake. Even the healthiest foods can lead to weight gain if consumed in quantities that exceed your body's needs.

2. **Calories and Goals:** The concept of eating according to your goals is crucial. For instance, eating a banana before a run provides quick energy, which is beneficial for performance.

However, consuming the same banana right before bed, when your body's caloric needs are lower, might contribute to unnecessary weight gain. Your body stores excess calories as fat, which is counterproductive if you're trying to manage your weight or achieve specific fitness goals.

3. **Timing and Context Matter:** It's not just about the quality of your food, but also the timing and context. A well-balanced meal eaten at the wrong time can hinder your progress. For instance, eating high-carb foods late at night might not be ideal for someone looking to lose weight or improve metabolic health. Similarly, consuming protein-heavy meals without adjusting for physical activity can lead to imbalanced nutrition.

4. **Aligning Diet with Personal Objectives:** Tailoring your diet to your specific goals—whether it's weight loss, muscle gain, or improved athletic performance—requires more than just choosing healthy foods. You need to consider the caloric content, nutrient timing, and how the foods fit into your overall daily intake. For instance, an athlete might need a higher carbohydrate intake around training sessions, while someone focused on weight loss might need to manage their caloric intake more strictly.

5. **Understanding Your Body's Needs:** Every individual has unique caloric and nutritional requirements based on their activity level, metabolism, and health goals. Eating healthy foods is just one part of the equation. The key is to understand how these foods fit into your daily caloric needs and to adjust portions and timing based on your personal objectives.

6. **The Bottom Line:** Eating healthy foods is important, but it's only part of the equation. To truly achieve your health and fitness goals, you need to consider not just what you eat but also how it aligns with your caloric needs and activity levels. By focusing on a well-rounded approach that includes proper timing and portion control, you can better tailor your diet to support your specific goals and achieve more effective results.

In conclusion, while eating healthy is a fundamental aspect of good nutrition, it's essential to tailor your diet to your individual goals and needs. Understanding how your food choices fit into your overall plan and making adjustments based on timing and caloric intake can help you achieve better outcomes and reach your health and fitness objectives more effectively.

# Losing Muscle or Losing Fat? Which Happens First?

When it comes to losing weight, one common question arises: do you lose muscle or fat first? The answer is that it depends on your diet, exercise routine, and overall energy balance. Understanding the body's energy pathways, especially during exercises like running 5 kilometers, can help explain how fat and muscle loss occur, and under what circumstances each might be prioritized.

## 1. Energy Pathways: How Your Body Uses Fuel

The body relies on different energy pathways depending on the type and intensity of exercise you perform. The two primary pathways are aerobic and anaerobic. These pathways dictate how your body burns fat or muscle for energy during exercise.

➤ **Aerobic Pathway**: This pathway is used during long-duration, low-to-moderate intensity exercise, such as jogging or running 5 kilometers at a steady pace. The body primarily relies on oxygen to produce energy in this state, using fat as the main source of fuel. This is where fat burning occurs because fat is broken down in the presence of oxygen to provide a continuous, long-lasting energy supply.

> **Anaerobic Pathway**: This pathway kicks in during short bursts of high-intensity activity, such as sprinting or lifting heavy weights. Since there's not enough time for oxygen to be utilized effectively, the body relies on glycogen (stored carbohydrates) for energy. This is a quicker but less efficient energy source, and it is less effective at burning fat. Over time, if glycogen stores are depleted, muscle tissue can also be broken down for energy, especially in a calorie-deficient state.

## 2. Muscle vs. Fat Loss: What Comes First?

> **When Diet is Poor or Protein is Lacking**: If your diet lacks sufficient protein or calories, your body may break down muscle tissue to meet energy demands. This is often the case in extreme calorie restriction or poorly designed diets. Muscle breakdown can happen first in these cases because muscle is metabolically expensive to maintain and provides a ready source of amino acids when the body is in need.

> **With Proper Nutrition and Strength Training**: If you maintain a proper diet with enough protein and engage in strength training alongside your cardio workouts, your body is more likely to preserve muscle mass and focus on burning fat. During aerobic activities like running 5 kilometers,

the body will primarily use fat as a fuel source if the intensity is moderate.

➤ **In Caloric Deficit**: To lose fat, you need to be in a caloric deficit, meaning you consume fewer calories than your body needs to maintain its current weight. With a balanced approach, fat loss can be prioritized over muscle loss. However, if the deficit is too extreme or prolonged without enough protein intake, muscle loss may occur.

## 3. Running 5 Kilometers: A Real-World Example

➤ **Aerobic State**: When you run 5 kilometers at a moderate, steady pace, your body is primarily relying on the aerobic energy pathway. As you run, your body uses oxygen to break down fats and carbohydrates, with a greater emphasis on burning fat the longer you run. This is why longer, steady-state cardio is associated with fat loss.

➤ **Anaerobic State**: If you perform high-intensity sprints during your run or increase the pace to a point where you are breathless, your body shifts into the anaerobic energy pathway. Here, glycogen stores are utilized to provide quick energy, and fat burning is minimized. Once glycogen stores are depleted, your body may even begin to break down muscle tissue if you're in a severe caloric deficit or don't consume enough protein.

## 4. How to Prioritize Fat Loss and Preserve Muscle

- ➤ **Adequate Protein Intake**: Ensuring your diet includes sufficient protein is key to preventing muscle loss. Aim for 1.6–2.2 grams of protein per kilogram of body weight, especially when in a calorie deficit.

- ➤ **Incorporating Strength Training**: Adding strength training to your routine can help signal your body to maintain muscle mass. This, combined with aerobic exercise, leads to more effective fat loss.

- ➤ **Moderate Caloric Deficit**: Avoid extreme calorie restriction, which can force your body into muscle breakdown for energy. A moderate deficit, coupled with proper nutrition, promotes fat loss while preserving muscle.

## 5. Conclusion: Muscle or Fat?

The type of energy pathway your body uses depends on the exercise intensity and duration. In general, aerobic activities like running at a moderate pace burn fat, while anaerobic activities focus on glycogen and can lead to muscle breakdown if you're not careful. To preserve muscle and prioritize fat loss, ensure you're eating enough protein, strength training regularly, and maintaining a balanced caloric deficit.

By understanding how your body uses fuel, you can create a workout and diet plan that helps you lose fat, preserve muscle, and achieve your fitness goals efficiently.

# Setting Realistic Goals for Fat Loss and Muscle Gain

When it comes to body transformation, it's essential to set achievable goals based on realistic expectations. For men, it's possible to lose 3-4% body fat per month, while women can aim for 2-3%. When it comes to muscle gain, males can optimally gain around 800 grams to 1.2 kilograms of muscle each month. But it's crucial to remember that muscle synthesis is a slow, steady process—dumping a bucket of water on a tree won't make it grow faster, and similarly, your body can't build muscle tissue any quicker than it can bio-synthesize efficiently.

## Gaining Weight: Fat, Water, or Muscle?

When the scale shows weight gain, it's not always muscle. Weight gain could be due to an increase in fat, water retention, or muscle. The body doesn't distinguish between the types of weight gain on the scale; what matters is the composition. Similarly, weight loss can also be a result of losing muscle, water, or fat, depending on how you approach your diet and training.

## The Order of Losing Weight: Muscle or Fat First?

Unfortunately, in many cases, muscle is often lost before fat. Muscle is a metabolically expensive tissue for the body to maintain—it requires more oxygen, blood flow, and nutrients. In times of caloric restriction, the body may view muscle as a burden and prioritize fat storage, especially since fat serves as an energy reserve that was essential during periods of famine or drought in human history. Fat is critical for survival, particularly during pregnancy, where the body will prioritize storing fat to support the growing embryo, even if the mother isn't eating sufficiently.

## Why Muscle Loss Happens First

When you cut calories or go on a diet without adequate resistance training, your body may break down muscle to meet its energy demands. This is because maintaining muscle requires significant resources. Without proper fuel and exercise to signal the body to keep its muscle mass, muscle is often the first to go. The body holds on to fat as a safeguard, a survival mechanism passed down through evolution.

## How to Preserve Muscle

The only way to preserve muscle during weight loss is through resistance training. When you perform resistance exercises, such as weightlifting, your muscles are signaled to stay, because they're still needed for work. Without this stimulus, muscle loss is almost inevitable in a caloric deficit. Resistance training, combined with sufficient protein intake, ensures that your body holds on to its muscle mass while burning fat for energy.

## Conclusion

Your body is not designed to rapidly gain muscle or lose fat without significant effort and the right approach. Muscle requires consistent resistance training and proper nutrition, while fat loss depends on creating a caloric deficit. Set realistic goals for both fat loss and muscle gain, and remember that the body has evolved to store fat as a survival mechanism. Resistance training is key to preserving muscle during weight loss, ensuring you achieve a balanced and sustainable transformation.

# The Science of Sleep:

Sleep is often an overlooked aspect of fitness, yet it plays a crucial role in muscle recovery, fat loss, and overall health. When you sleep, your body is not just resting but actively working to repair tissues, build muscles, and regulate key hormones like cortisol and growth hormone, which directly impact fat storage and muscle growth. During deep sleep, growth hormone peaks, helping to repair muscle fibers that were broken down during exercise. This is why getting quality sleep is just as important as a solid workout and nutrition plan.

On the other hand, a lack of sleep can derail your fitness goals. Studies have shown that people who sleep fewer hours tend to consume more calories and store more fat. This is because inadequate sleep increases levels of ghrelin (the hunger hormone) and decreases leptin (the hormone that signals fullness). As a result, even if your diet and exercise are on point, sleep deprivation can still slow down fat loss or even lead to weight gain. Moreover, your body becomes more resistant to insulin, which makes it harder to burn fat and can increase the risk of diabetes.

## Importance of Sleep Cycles for Optimal Performance:

Sleep is divided into multiple cycles, primarily consisting of REM (Rapid Eye Movement) and NREM (Non-REM) stages. Each cycle plays a vital role in physical and mental recovery. The deep stages of NREM sleep are where most of the body's healing and muscle repair happen, while REM sleep supports brain function, mood regulation, and motor skill learning.

When you miss out on these cycles, you not only compromise your mental focus and emotional resilience but also reduce your body's ability to repair muscles and burn fat efficiently. For example, athletes or regular gym-goers who don't get enough sleep may find it harder to progress in their training. Even a slight deficit in sleep can lead to reduced strength, slower reaction times, and poor endurance.

To ensure optimal performance, aim for 7-9 hours of sleep per night. Sticking to a consistent sleep schedule—going to bed and waking up at the same time every day—can help regulate your body's internal clock and improve the quality of your sleep cycles.

## Techniques for Improving Sleep Quality:

Improving sleep quality doesn't require drastic lifestyle changes. Instead, adopting a few habits can lead to better sleep and, subsequently, better fitness results:

1. **Limit Screen Time Before Bed**: Blue light from screens can interfere with melatonin production, the hormone that signals it's time to sleep. Turn off electronics at least 30 minutes before bed.

2. **Create a Sleep-Inducing Environment**: A dark, cool, and quiet room is the best setup for sleep. Consider blackout curtains, earplugs, or a white noise machine to help block distractions.

3. **Practice Relaxation Techniques**: Meditation, deep breathing exercises, or even light stretching before bed can help calm the nervous system and prepare your body for restful sleep.

4. **Limit Caffeine and Heavy Meals**: Caffeine can stay in your system for up to 8 hours, so avoid it late in the day. Similarly, large meals before bed can disrupt digestion and affect sleep.

5. **Exercise Regularly**: Regular physical activity, especially earlier in the day, can improve sleep quality. However, avoid vigorous exercise right before bed as it can leave you too energized to fall asleep.

By prioritizing sleep and following these techniques, you can dramatically improve your body's ability to recover, burn fat, and build muscle. Sleep isn't just downtime; it's an essential component of any successful fitness journey.

# Mind-Body Connection in Fitness:

When it comes to fitness, the mind often plays as crucial a role as the body. While it's easy to focus on physical aspects like lifting weights, running, or maintaining proper form, the mental side of fitness is just as vital for success. The connection between the mind and body can either enhance or hinder your progress, depending on how well you leverage it. Whether you're trying to lose weight, build muscle, or improve endurance, mental focus and discipline are key factors in achieving your goals.

## The Role of Mental Focus and Discipline in Achieving Fitness Goals:

Mental focus in fitness refers to the ability to concentrate on your workout and push through discomfort, fatigue, or distractions. Discipline involves consistently following a workout routine and adhering to healthy habits over time, even when motivation is low. Together, mental focus and discipline create a powerful foundation for long-term fitness success.

For example, during a difficult workout, your mind often gives up before your body truly reaches its limits. Those who master mental focus can push past the initial feelings of discomfort or fatigue, accessing the extra strength or endurance needed to complete challenging sets or run that extra mile. On the other hand, a lack of focus may lead to cutting corners, skipping reps, or finishing a workout prematurely, which can stall progress.

Discipline, on the other hand, is the force that keeps you on track over the long haul. Motivation comes and goes, but discipline keeps you moving forward. It's about showing up to the gym even when you don't feel like it, preparing your meals even when you're tired, and staying consistent with your goals. By building mental discipline, you set yourself up for incremental, steady progress that eventually leads to massive changes over time.

## Benefits of Meditation, Visualization, and Mindfulness in Workouts:

Incorporating mindfulness practices such as meditation, visualization, and mindfulness into your fitness routine can significantly enhance both mental and physical performance.

1. **Meditation**: Regular meditation can help improve focus, reduce stress, and enhance overall mental clarity. When applied to fitness, meditation allows you to tune into your body and stay present during your workouts. It can also improve your

relationship with exercise, helping you appreciate the process rather than solely focusing on the outcome. Additionally, meditation can aid in recovery by lowering cortisol levels (the stress hormone), which promotes better rest and muscle repair.

2. **Visualization**: This technique involves mentally rehearsing a workout or a specific goal before you actually perform it. Visualization has been used by top athletes for decades to improve performance. For example, before lifting a heavy weight, you can visualize yourself completing the lift with perfect form. This mental rehearsal primes your brain and body to execute the movement more effectively, increasing your chances of success. Visualization also helps set clear, achievable goals by creating a mental image of what you want to accomplish, whether it's a new personal best or reaching a certain fitness milestone.

3. **Mindfulness**: Being mindful during workouts means being fully aware of your body, your movements, and your breath. When you practice mindfulness, you focus on every rep, every step, and every breath, which not only improves your performance but also helps prevent injury. Mindfulness helps you listen to your body's cues—whether you're overexerting or need to

adjust your form—and respond accordingly. This can help enhance the quality of your workouts, making each movement more effective.

Furthermore, mindfulness has a profound impact on managing stress and anxiety, which can negatively affect workout performance and recovery. By staying present and avoiding distractions, you can also improve mental toughness, helping you power through difficult exercises or resist temptations like skipping workouts or indulging in unhealthy food.

## Bridging the Mind-Body Gap for Optimal Fitness:

Bringing mental focus, discipline, and mindfulness together creates a holistic approach to fitness. This mind-body connection goes beyond just getting through a workout; it allows you to fully engage with the process, making exercise a more enriching and sustainable part of your life.

Here are a few strategies to bridge the mind-body gap in fitness:

➤ **Set clear, achievable goals**: Visualization works best when you know exactly what you want to achieve. Break your larger goals into smaller, more manageable ones, and visualize yourself succeeding step by step.

> **Incorporate mindfulness in every session**: Pay attention to how your body moves and feels during every exercise. Engage your muscles deliberately, focus on your breath, and tune into your body's feedback.

> **Practice mental resilience**: Push through mental barriers by building a mindset that embraces challenges and discomfort. Every time you overcome an obstacle, you're strengthening your mind as much as your body.

In conclusion, the mind-body connection is a powerful tool in achieving fitness goals. By developing mental focus and discipline, and integrating meditation, visualization, and mindfulness into your fitness routine, you not only improve your workouts but also create lasting change in both your physical and mental well-being.

# The Role of Hormones in Fitness:

Hormones are chemical messengers that regulate many of the body's essential processes, including fat loss, muscle gain, and metabolism. When it comes to fitness, a few key hormones—testosterone, cortisol, insulin, and growth hormone—play a significant role in shaping your progress. Understanding how these hormones function can help you optimize your workouts, nutrition, and recovery to achieve better results.

## 1. Testosterone: The Muscle-Building Hormone

Testosterone is often referred to as the "muscle-building" hormone due to its crucial role in muscle growth, repair, and fat loss. Both men and women produce testosterone, though men typically have much higher levels, which is why they generally build muscle more easily.

➤ **Muscle Gain**: Testosterone promotes protein synthesis, the process where your body builds muscle tissue. It also increases the production of red blood cells, which helps deliver oxygen to muscles during exercise, improving performance and endurance.

> **Fat Loss**: Testosterone helps regulate fat distribution in the body. Higher levels of testosterone are associated with a lower body fat percentage, while low testosterone levels can lead to fat gain, especially around the abdominal area.

> **Recovery**: Testosterone aids in faster muscle recovery by repairing muscle fibers damaged during workouts. This allows for more intense and frequent training sessions, leading to faster muscle gains.

To boost testosterone naturally, focus on strength training exercises that engage large muscle groups, such as squats and deadlifts. Additionally, proper sleep, stress management, and a balanced diet rich in healthy fats (like avocados and nuts) can help maintain healthy testosterone levels.

## 2. Cortisol: The Stress Hormone

Cortisol is often referred to as the "stress hormone" because it is released in response to physical or emotional stress. While cortisol is essential for regulating energy and managing stress, chronically elevated levels can hinder your fitness progress.

> **Muscle Breakdown**: High levels of cortisol can lead to muscle breakdown, as it promotes the breakdown of proteins into amino acids to be used

for energy. This is especially problematic when cortisol remains elevated for extended periods, such as during chronic stress or overtraining.

➤ **Fat Storage**: Cortisol is linked to fat storage, particularly in the abdominal area. This is because cortisol increases insulin resistance, making it harder for your body to process glucose. As a result, excess glucose is stored as fat.

➤ **Energy Regulation**: Cortisol helps regulate energy levels by releasing glucose into the bloodstream, providing a quick energy boost. However, if cortisol levels remain too high, it can lead to energy crashes and fatigue, making it difficult to maintain a consistent workout routine.

To manage cortisol levels, it's important to incorporate stress-reducing activities like meditation, yoga, and adequate rest into your routine. Avoid overtraining by allowing sufficient recovery time between workouts and ensuring proper nutrition to fuel your body.

## 3. Insulin: The Blood Sugar Regulator

Insulin is a hormone produced by the pancreas that regulates blood sugar levels. It plays a critical role in how your body stores and uses energy from food, particularly carbohydrates. While insulin is essential for muscle growth, improper insulin management can lead to fat gain.

- **Muscle Growth**: Insulin promotes the uptake of glucose and amino acids into muscle cells, which is essential for muscle repair and growth. After a workout, insulin helps shuttle nutrients into your muscles, making it a key player in post-workout recovery.

- **Fat Storage**: When insulin levels are chronically elevated (often due to a high-sugar diet), the body becomes more efficient at storing fat. Excess glucose that isn't used for energy is stored as fat, leading to weight gain and insulin resistance over time.

- **Metabolism**: Insulin affects your metabolism by controlling how your body uses carbohydrates, fats, and proteins. Balanced insulin levels help maintain stable energy levels, while insulin spikes (due to eating high-sugar or processed foods) can lead to energy crashes and increased fat storage.

To optimize insulin function, focus on a balanced diet with whole foods, complex carbohydrates, and lean proteins. Avoid excessive sugar and refined carbohydrates, and time your carb intake around workouts to replenish muscle glycogen stores.

## 4. Growth Hormone: The Recovery and Fat-Burning Hormone

Growth hormone (GH), produced by the pituitary gland, is essential for tissue growth, cell repair, and fat metabolism. It plays a significant role in muscle recovery, fat loss, and maintaining overall body composition.

- **Muscle Growth and Repair**: Growth hormone stimulates protein synthesis, helping to build and repair muscle tissue. It also enhances the body's ability to use amino acids to create new muscle fibers, making it vital for recovery after intense workouts.

- **Fat Loss**: GH increases lipolysis, the breakdown of fats into fatty acids, which are then used as energy. This makes growth hormone an important hormone for fat loss, especially when combined with strength training and high-intensity exercise.

- **Cell Regeneration**: GH promotes the regeneration of cells, tissues, and bones, making it essential for overall health and fitness. It also improves collagen synthesis, which is important for joint and tendon health.

Growth hormone levels naturally decline with age, but you can boost GH production through activities like high-intensity interval training (HIIT), strength training, and getting adequate sleep. Deep sleep, particularly during slow-wave sleep, is when growth hormone production peaks.

## Optimizing Hormonal Balance for Fitness:

To achieve your fitness goals, it's essential to maintain a balance of these hormones. Here are some practical tips:

- **Strength Training**: Lifting weights stimulates testosterone and growth hormone production, helping with muscle growth and fat loss.

- **Adequate Sleep**: Sleep is critical for regulating hormones like cortisol and growth hormone. Aim for 7-9 hours of quality sleep each night.

- **Balanced Diet**: Include a mix of proteins, healthy fats, and complex carbs to stabilize insulin and promote hormone balance.

- **Stress Management**: Incorporate mindfulness practices, yoga, or other relaxation techniques to keep cortisol in check.

- **Proper Recovery**: Allow time for your body to rest and recover between workouts to avoid overtraining and elevated cortisol levels.

In conclusion, hormones like testosterone, cortisol, insulin, and growth hormone play pivotal roles in your fitness journey. By understanding how they influence muscle growth, fat loss, and metabolism, you can tailor your exercise, nutrition, and recovery strategies for optimal results.

# Gut Health and Fitness:

The gut, often referred to as the "second brain," plays a crucial role in overall health, particularly in relation to fitness. The gut microbiome, a collection of trillions of bacteria and microorganisms in the digestive tract, has a profound impact on metabolism, immunity, and body composition. An unhealthy gut can hinder your progress in fat loss, muscle gain, and overall well-being, while a healthy gut can enhance your performance and recovery.

## Exploring the Gut Microbiome and Its Relationship with Fitness

1. **Metabolism and Weight Management**: The gut microbiome is heavily involved in how the body processes and stores fat, as well as how it regulates appetite. Research shows that certain bacteria in the gut can influence weight gain or loss. An imbalance in the microbiome, known as dysbiosis, can slow metabolism and increase fat storage.

   - **Fat Storage**: Some gut bacteria are more efficient at extracting energy (calories) from food, which can contribute to weight gain. Conversely, a healthy gut microbiome supports the proper breakdown and absorption of nutrients, helping to maintain a healthy weight.

- **Appetite Regulation**: The gut produces various hormones that influence hunger, such as ghrelin (the hunger hormone) and leptin (the satiety hormone). A balanced gut helps regulate these hormones, reducing the likelihood of overeating or cravings.

2. **Immunity**: About 70-80% of the immune system resides in the gut. The microbiome acts as a barrier against harmful pathogens while helping to regulate immune responses. A healthy gut can prevent chronic inflammation, which is a common obstacle to fitness progress.

- **Reduced Inflammation**: Inflammation can lead to muscle soreness, fatigue, and slower recovery times. A balanced gut microbiome promotes anti-inflammatory responses, which can help reduce soreness and support faster muscle recovery.

- **Immune Support**: For athletes or those regularly exercising, maintaining a strong immune system is vital to prevent illness, which can disrupt training routines. A healthy gut boosts immunity and keeps the body more resilient.

3.  **Body Composition**: The gut microbiome also plays a role in body composition, influencing fat storage and muscle mass. Studies suggest that a diverse microbiome is linked to lower body fat and better muscle tone. Certain gut bacteria are associated with improved fat oxidation and increased lean muscle mass.

    - **Muscle Mass**: A healthy gut may help with better protein absorption, which is critical for muscle repair and growth. Additionally, some gut bacteria produce short-chain fatty acids (SCFAs) that support energy production and fat loss, further contributing to improved body composition.

    - **Fat Loss**: Gut health affects how efficiently your body uses fat for energy. A balanced microbiome helps with the regulation of insulin and blood sugar levels, reducing fat storage and promoting fat loss.

## Foods That Promote Gut Health

To support gut health and enhance fitness performance, incorporating gut-friendly foods into your diet is essential. These foods help nourish beneficial bacteria and contribute to a more balanced and diverse microbiome.

1.  **Probiotic-Rich Foods**: Probiotics are live bacteria that can enhance the gut microbiome by increasing the population of beneficial bacteria. Consuming foods rich in probiotics helps maintain a healthy balance and supports digestion.

    *   **Yogurt**: Yogurt is one of the most common probiotic-rich foods, containing strains like *Lactobacillus* and *Bifidobacterium*, which support gut health. Choose unsweetened, plain varieties for maximum benefit.

    *   **Kefir**: A fermented milk drink, kefir is rich in probiotics and more potent than yogurt due to its diverse bacterial profile.

    *   **Sauerkraut and Kimchi**: These fermented vegetables are loaded with probiotics and also offer the added benefits of fiber, which is crucial for gut health.

2.  **Prebiotic Foods**: Prebiotics are types of fiber that feed the beneficial bacteria in the gut, allowing them to thrive. Incorporating prebiotic-rich foods helps to improve digestion and gut health.

    *   **Garlic and Onions**: Both are rich in inulin, a type of prebiotic fiber that promotes the growth of beneficial bacteria.

- **Bananas**: A simple and accessible source of prebiotics, bananas help balance the bacteria in your gut and improve digestion.

- **Asparagus and Jerusalem Artichokes**: These vegetables are high in prebiotic fibers, which foster a healthy microbiome.

3. **High-Fiber Foods**: Fiber plays an essential role in gut health by promoting regular bowel movements and preventing constipation. It also serves as food for the beneficial bacteria in the gut, helping to maintain a healthy balance.

   - **Whole Grains**: Brown rice, oats, quinoa, and whole wheat are all high in fiber, promoting better digestion and overall gut health.

   - **Leafy Greens**: Spinach, kale, and Swiss chard provide fiber and other nutrients that feed gut bacteria and support digestion.

   - **Legumes**: Beans, lentils, and chickpeas are excellent sources of fiber, helping to maintain a diverse and healthy gut microbiome.

4. **Polyphenol-Rich Foods**: Polyphenols are compounds found in plant-based foods that have antioxidant properties and support gut health by promoting the growth of beneficial bacteria.

- **Green Tea**: Rich in polyphenols, green tea can help promote the growth of healthy gut bacteria and reduce harmful ones.

- **Berries**: Blueberries, raspberries, and strawberries are packed with polyphenols that have a positive impact on gut bacteria and overall health.

- **Dark Chocolate**: In moderation, dark chocolate is a good source of polyphenols that can boost the diversity of gut bacteria.

5. **Omega-3 Fatty Acids**: Omega-3 fatty acids, found in foods like fatty fish (salmon, mackerel, sardines), flaxseeds, and walnuts, have anti-inflammatory properties that support gut health and reduce inflammation in the body.

## Tips for Maintaining Gut Health for Optimal Fitness:

- **Diverse Diet**: Eat a wide variety of foods to ensure your microbiome remains diverse. Different types of bacteria thrive on different nutrients, so incorporating a range of fruits, vegetables, grains, and proteins helps maintain a healthy gut.

- **Hydration**: Drinking enough water is essential for maintaining a healthy digestive system and supporting the gut. Proper hydration helps with nutrient absorption and regular bowel movements.

> **Avoid Processed Foods**: Processed and sugary foods can feed harmful bacteria and lead to an imbalance in the microbiome. Focus on whole, natural foods for optimal gut health.

> **Limit Antibiotic Use**: While antibiotics can be necessary for treating infections, overuse can harm the gut by killing both harmful and beneficial bacteria. Always consult a doctor before taking antibiotics.

In conclusion, gut health is deeply intertwined with fitness, affecting metabolism, immunity, and body composition. By prioritizing a gut-friendly diet rich in probiotics, prebiotics, fiber, polyphenols, and omega-3s, you can support your overall fitness goals and enhance your body's ability to recover, perform, and maintain a healthy weight.

# Cardiovascular Training vs. Resistance Training:

When it comes to fitness, cardiovascular training and resistance training are two fundamental approaches, each with its distinct benefits and downsides. Understanding these differences is crucial for tailoring your workout routine to meet specific goals, whether they involve improving heart health, building muscle, or achieving overall fitness.

## Cardiovascular Training

**Cardiovascular training**, often referred to as aerobic exercise, involves activities that increase your heart rate and breathing for an extended period. This type of exercise primarily aims to enhance the efficiency of the cardiovascular system and improve overall endurance. Examples include running, cycling, swimming, and brisk walking.

## Benefits:

1. **Improved Heart Health**: Cardiovascular exercise strengthens the heart muscle, improving its ability to pump blood efficiently. This leads to better circulation and reduced risk of heart disease. Regular aerobic exercise helps lower blood

pressure, reduce cholesterol levels, and enhance overall cardiovascular function.

2. **Enhanced Endurance**: By engaging in aerobic activities, you increase your stamina and endurance. This not only helps with daily activities but also improves performance in other types of exercise and sports. Increased endurance means you can sustain physical activity for longer periods without experiencing fatigue.

3. **Calorie Burning and Weight Management**: Cardiovascular training is effective for burning calories and managing body weight. Activities like running or cycling can burn a significant number of calories, which, when combined with a balanced diet, supports weight loss and maintenance. Regular aerobic exercise helps create a caloric deficit, leading to fat loss.

4. **Improved Respiratory Function**: Engaging in cardiovascular exercises enhances lung capacity and efficiency. This improves oxygen intake and utilization, contributing to better overall respiratory health. Enhanced lung function supports higher exercise intensity and recovery.

5. **Mental Health Benefits**: Aerobic exercise is known to release endorphins, which are natural mood lifters. Regular cardiovascular training can

help reduce symptoms of anxiety, depression, and stress. The "runner's high" is a well-documented phenomenon where individuals experience elevated mood and mental clarity post-exercise.

## Downsides:

1. **Potential for Overuse Injuries**: Prolonged or excessive cardiovascular exercise, especially high-impact activities like running, can lead to overuse injuries such as shin splints, stress fractures, and joint pain. It's essential to balance aerobic workouts with rest and recovery to prevent these issues.

2. **Muscle Loss**: While cardiovascular exercise is excellent for fat loss, excessive cardio without adequate resistance training can lead to muscle loss. The body may break down muscle tissue for energy if it is not provided with sufficient resistance exercises.

3. **Limited Muscle Strength and Growth**: Cardiovascular training primarily focuses on endurance and does not significantly contribute to muscle strength or growth. For those aiming to build muscle mass or increase strength, aerobic exercise alone will not suffice.

4. **Time-Consuming**: Effective cardiovascular workouts often require a longer duration

to achieve significant benefits, which can be challenging for those with busy schedules. To see substantial improvements in endurance and fitness, individuals may need to dedicate more time to cardio exercises.

## Resistance Training

**Resistance training**, also known as strength training or weight training, involves exercises that work against resistance to build muscle strength and endurance. This can include lifting weights, using resistance bands, or performing bodyweight exercises like push-ups and squats.

## Benefits:

1. **Muscle Strength and Growth**: Resistance training is highly effective for increasing muscle strength, size, and definition. By challenging muscles with progressive overload, you stimulate muscle growth and improve overall strength. This type of training enhances functional strength, which is beneficial for everyday activities and overall fitness.

2. **Improved Metabolism**: Building muscle through resistance training increases your basal metabolic rate (BMR), which means you burn more calories at rest. This contributes to better weight

management and fat loss over time. Muscle tissue is metabolically active, requiring more energy to maintain than fat tissue.

3. **Bone Health**: Resistance training improves bone density and reduces the risk of osteoporosis. Weight-bearing exercises help stimulate bone growth and strength, which is particularly important for older adults to prevent bone loss and fractures.

4. **Enhanced Functional Fitness**: Strength training improves functional fitness by enhancing the ability to perform daily tasks with ease. Activities like lifting groceries, climbing stairs, or carrying heavy objects become easier as your strength and endurance improve.

5. **Injury Prevention**: By strengthening muscles, tendons, and ligaments, resistance training helps protect against injuries. Stronger muscles support and stabilize joints, reducing the risk of strains, sprains, and other common injuries.

Downsides:

1. **Risk of Injury**: Improper technique or excessive weight can lead to injuries such as strains, sprains, and joint issues. It's crucial to use proper form,

start with appropriate weights, and gradually increase resistance to minimize the risk of injury.

2. **Limited Cardiovascular Benefits**: While resistance training improves muscle strength and metabolism, it does not significantly enhance cardiovascular endurance. For overall fitness, resistance training should be complemented with cardiovascular exercise.

3. **Plateaus in Progress**: Progress in resistance training can sometimes stall, leading to plateaus where muscle growth or strength gains become stagnant. To continue making progress, individuals need to vary their workouts, increase weights, or adjust training techniques.

4. **Equipment and Space Requirements**: Effective resistance training often requires access to equipment such as weights, resistance bands, or machines. This may not always be feasible in home settings without a well-equipped gym or sufficient space.

## When to Prioritize One Over the Other

**Cardiovascular Training:**

➤ **For Weight Loss**: If your primary goal is to burn calories and reduce body fat, prioritize cardiovascular exercise. It's effective for creating a caloric deficit and improving overall endurance.

➤ **For Cardiovascular Health**: To improve heart and lung function, cardiovascular training should be a priority. Regular aerobic exercise supports cardiovascular health and reduces the risk of heart disease.

➤ **For Mental Health**: If you seek to reduce stress, anxiety, or depression, cardiovascular exercise is beneficial due to its mood-lifting effects and endorphin release.

**Resistance Training**:

➤ **For Muscle Building**: If your goal is to increase muscle mass, strength, and definition, focus on resistance training. It's the most effective way to build and maintain muscle.

➤ **For Metabolic Boost**: To enhance your metabolism and support long-term weight management, incorporate resistance training into your routine. Building muscle increases your BMR and aids in fat loss.

➤ **For Functional Fitness and Injury Prevention**: If you want to improve your ability to perform daily tasks and reduce the risk of injury, prioritize resistance training. Stronger muscles and bones support better functional fitness and overall physical health.

**Balanced Approach**: For optimal results, a balanced approach incorporating both cardiovascular and resistance training is recommended. Combining these forms of exercise ensures comprehensive fitness benefits, including improved endurance, strength, metabolism, and overall health. Tailor your workout plan to your specific goals, and consider integrating both types of training to achieve a well-rounded fitness regimen.

## Importance of Hydration

## How Water Affects Metabolism, Performance, and Recovery

**Metabolism and Water:** Water is essential for various metabolic processes in the body. It aids in the digestion and absorption of nutrients, ensures the proper function of enzymes, and facilitates the transport of nutrients to cells. Adequate hydration helps maintain an optimal balance of electrolytes and supports cellular functions. Without enough water, the body's metabolic processes can become inefficient, leading to reduced energy levels and impaired performance.

**Performance and Hydration:** Hydration significantly impacts athletic performance. Water helps regulate body temperature through sweating and respiration. During exercise, the body loses water through sweat, and if this loss is not replenished, it can lead to dehydration. Dehydration negatively affects endurance, strength, and overall exercise performance. Symptoms of dehydration include fatigue, reduced strength, decreased coordination, and slower reaction times. Staying hydrated ensures that the cardiovascular system functions efficiently, allowing for better oxygen delivery to muscles and improved exercise performance.

**Recovery and Hydration:** Post-exercise hydration is crucial for recovery. Water helps in the replenishment of lost fluids and electrolytes, which aids in muscle repair and reduces the risk of cramps and injuries. Proper hydration helps flush out metabolic waste products generated during exercise and supports the repair and rebuilding of muscle tissue. Drinking enough water post-workout also helps restore optimal blood volume and reduces the risk of post-exercise fatigue.

## Hydration Strategies for Optimal Health and Fitness

1. **Establish a Hydration Routine:** Developing a regular hydration routine helps maintain consistent fluid intake. Aim to drink water throughout the day rather than consuming large

quantities at once. A good starting point is to drink at least 8-10 glasses of water daily, but this amount can vary based on individual needs, activity levels, and environmental conditions.

2. **Pre-Hydrate:** Before engaging in physical activity, ensure you are adequately hydrated. Drinking water in the hours leading up to exercise can help maintain fluid balance and optimize performance. For intense workouts or prolonged exercise sessions, consider drinking electrolyte-enriched beverages to replace lost minerals.

3. **Monitor Hydration Status:** Pay attention to signs of dehydration, such as dark urine, dry mouth, and fatigue. Using a hydration tracker or simply monitoring your urine color can be effective indicators of your hydration status. Ideally, urine should be light yellow.

4. **Hydrate During Exercise:** During prolonged or intense exercise, consume water regularly to prevent dehydration. For workouts lasting longer than an hour, consider incorporating sports drinks that contain electrolytes to replenish sodium, potassium, and other essential minerals.

5. **Post-Exercise Rehydration:** After exercise, focus on replenishing lost fluids and electrolytes. Drinking water is crucial, but for longer or more

intense workouts, combining water with a source of carbohydrates and electrolytes can further enhance recovery.

6. **Adapt to Environmental Conditions:** In hot and humid conditions, your body loses more water through sweat. Increase your fluid intake to match the increased loss. Conversely, in cold environments, you may still lose water through increased respiratory loss, so maintain regular hydration habits.

7. **Include Hydrating Foods:** Incorporate water-rich foods into your diet, such as fruits and vegetables (e.g., watermelon, cucumbers, oranges). These foods contribute to your overall fluid intake and provide additional nutrients beneficial for health and performance.

8. **Avoid Excessive Caffeine and Alcohol:** Both caffeine and alcohol can have diuretic effects, leading to increased fluid loss. While moderate consumption is generally acceptable, excessive intake of these substances should be balanced with increased water consumption.

By following these hydration strategies, you can support optimal metabolism, enhance performance, and promote effective recovery, contributing to overall health and fitness.

# Fitness for Different Life Stages

Fitness needs evolve significantly across the different stages of life. As we age, our bodies undergo various changes that necessitate adjustments in our exercise routines and overall approach to fitness. Understanding how these changes affect our physical health and tailoring exercise programs accordingly can help optimize well-being at every stage of life.

## Fitness Needs Across Various Ages

### Teens (13-19 Years Old):

1. **Growth and Development:** During adolescence, individuals experience rapid growth and hormonal changes. Fitness routines for teens should focus on developing fundamental movement skills, building strength, and enhancing cardiovascular fitness. Activities should be diverse and engaging to encourage lifelong habits.

2. **Bone Health:** Weight-bearing exercises such as running, jumping, and resistance training are crucial for bone development. These activities help increase bone density and reduce the risk of osteoporosis later in life.

3. **Skill Development:** Teens should engage in activities that improve coordination, balance, and agility. Sports, gymnastics, and dance are

excellent options that combine fitness with skill development.

4. **Mental Health:** Exercise during adolescence can help manage stress, improve mood, and support mental health. Engaging in regular physical activity can contribute to better academic performance and overall well-being.

## 20s:

1. **Peak Physical Performance:** In their 20s, individuals are often at their peak physical performance. This is a great time to focus on building strength, endurance, and flexibility. Incorporate a mix of cardio, resistance training, and flexibility exercises to maximize fitness.

2. **Establishing Habits:** Developing a consistent exercise routine during this decade sets the foundation for lifelong fitness. Establishing healthy habits now can prevent weight gain and support metabolic health as one ages.

3. **Preventive Fitness:** Preventive measures such as maintaining a healthy weight, reducing stress, and avoiding excessive alcohol and tobacco use are important. Engaging in regular exercise helps mitigate the risk of chronic diseases such as heart disease and diabetes.

4. **Fitness for Career Demands:** Depending on career demands, incorporate exercises that counteract sedentary behaviors, such as desk jobs. Strength training and stretching can help alleviate the effects of prolonged sitting and improve posture.

**40s:**

1. **Managing Metabolism:** As metabolism begins to slow down, it's important to focus on a balanced exercise routine that includes both cardio and strength training. Strength training helps counteract muscle loss and maintain a healthy metabolism.

2. **Joint Health:** Joint health becomes more significant in the 40s. Low-impact exercises such as swimming, cycling, and using elliptical machines can reduce stress on joints while still providing effective cardiovascular workouts.

3. **Stress and Work-Life Balance:** Balancing fitness with career and family responsibilities is crucial. Incorporate time-efficient workouts, such as high-intensity interval training (HIIT) or circuit training, to achieve maximum results in shorter periods.

4. **Health Conditions:** Address any emerging health conditions, such as hypertension or high cholesterol, through appropriate exercise and

lifestyle modifications. Consult with healthcare professionals to tailor exercise programs to individual health needs.

**Seniors (65+ Years Old):**

1. **Maintaining Mobility:** For seniors, the primary focus should be on maintaining mobility, flexibility, and balance. Activities such as walking, stretching, and balance exercises can help prevent falls and improve overall quality of life.

2. **Strength Training:** Strength training remains important to preserve muscle mass and bone density. Light weights or resistance bands can be used to perform exercises that target major muscle groups.

3. **Cardiovascular Health:** Low-impact cardiovascular exercises, such as walking, swimming, or cycling, are ideal for maintaining heart health without putting excessive strain on the body.

4. **Adapted Exercises:** Adapt exercises to accommodate any physical limitations or chronic conditions. Exercises should be tailored to individual capabilities and performed at a comfortable intensity.

5. **Social Engagement:** Participating in group fitness classes or community activities can provide social interaction and motivation, which are important for mental and emotional well-being.

## Tailoring Exercise Routines Based on Age, Body Changes, and Health Conditions

**Teens:**

- **Focus:** Skill development, bone health, and overall fitness.

- **Types of Exercises:** Sports, weight-bearing activities, agility drills, and flexibility exercises.

- **Considerations:** Ensure activities are enjoyable and diverse to foster a lifelong commitment to fitness.

## 20s:

- **Focus:** Building strength, endurance, and establishing long-term habits.

- **Types of Exercises:** Resistance training, cardio, flexibility routines, and recreational sports.

- **Considerations:** Prioritize a balanced approach to fitness and address career-related physical challenges.

## 40s:

- **Focus:** Managing metabolism, joint health, and balancing fitness with life demands.

- **Types of Exercises:** Strength training, low-impact cardio, stretching, and flexibility exercises.

> **Considerations:** Adapt workouts to accommodate changes in metabolism and potential joint issues.

**Seniors:**

> **Focus:** Maintaining mobility, strength, balance, and overall health.

> **Types of Exercises:** Low-impact cardio, strength training with light weights or resistance bands, balance exercises, and stretching.

> **Considerations:** Modify exercises to fit physical limitations, and consider social aspects of fitness.

Understanding how fitness needs change with age and body changes allows for the development of personalized exercise routines that support overall health and well-being throughout life. By adapting fitness programs to meet the specific needs of each life stage, individuals can maintain optimal health and enjoy a higher quality of life

## Supplements: What Works and What Doesn't

Supplements are widely used in the fitness and health industry to support various goals, from muscle growth to fat loss. However, not all supplements offer the benefits they claim, and their effectiveness can vary based on individual needs and goals. Understanding what works and what doesn't can help make informed decisions about supplement use. This section provides an analysis of popular supplements and offers guidance on their effective use.

## Popular Supplements and Their Efficacy

### 1. Protein Powder

**Purpose:** Protein powder is commonly used to increase protein intake, which is essential for muscle repair, growth, and overall recovery.

**Types:**

➢ **Whey Protein:** A complete protein derived from milk, quickly absorbed, and rich in essential amino acids.

➢ **Casein Protein:** Also from milk but digested more slowly, providing a steady release of amino acids.

➢ **Plant-Based Proteins:** Derived from sources such as peas, rice, and hemp, suitable for vegetarians and those with dairy allergies.

**Effectiveness:**

➢ **Muscle Growth:** Protein powder can support muscle growth and repair when combined with resistance training. It helps meet daily protein needs, particularly when dietary intake is insufficient.

➢ **Recovery:** Consuming protein post-workout can aid in muscle recovery and reduce muscle soreness.

## Usage:

➢ **Timing:** Optimal protein intake is often spread throughout the day, with a focus on post-workout consumption to maximize recovery.

➢ **Dosage:** Generally, 20-30 grams per serving is effective. Adjust based on individual protein needs and overall dietary intake.

### 2. Creatine

**Purpose:** Creatine is a naturally occurring compound that helps supply energy to muscle cells, enhancing strength, power, and muscle mass.

## Types:

➢ **Creatine Monohydrate:** The most studied and commonly used form of creatine.

➢ **Creatine Ethyl Ester, Buffered Creatine:** Variants that claim to offer better absorption or fewer side effects, though evidence is mixed.

## Effectiveness:

➢ **Strength and Power:** Creatine is well-supported by research for improving strength, power, and performance in high-intensity, short-duration activities like weightlifting and sprinting.

➢ **Muscle Mass:** It can contribute to muscle growth due to increased water retention in muscle cells and enhanced protein synthesis.

**Usage:**

- **Loading Phase:** Optional 20 grams per day (split into 4 doses) for 5-7 days, followed by a maintenance dose of 3-5 grams per day.

- **Continuous Use:** A consistent daily dose of 3-5 grams can be effective without the loading phase.

## 3. Branched-Chain Amino Acids (BCAAs)

**Purpose:** BCAAs (leucine, isoleucine, valine) are essential amino acids that play a role in muscle protein synthesis and energy production.

**Effectiveness:**

- **Muscle Recovery:** BCAAs may help reduce muscle soreness and improve recovery, particularly when consumed before or during exercise.

- **Exercise Performance:** Some studies suggest BCAAs can reduce fatigue during prolonged exercise, though the impact may be modest compared to whole protein sources.

**Usage:**

- **Dosage:** Typically 5-10 grams before or during exercise. The benefits are often more pronounced if dietary protein is insufficient.

### 4.  Fat Burners

**Purpose:** Fat burners claim to enhance fat loss by increasing metabolism, suppressing appetite, or improving fat oxidation.

**Common Ingredients:**

➤ **Caffeine:** A well-known stimulant that can increase metabolic rate and improve exercise performance.

➤ **Green Tea Extract:** Contains compounds that may support fat oxidation.

➤ **Yohimbine:** A stimulant that may help with fat loss, though side effects are possible.

**Effectiveness:**

➤ **Short-Term Effects:** Some fat burners can provide a modest boost to metabolism and energy expenditure. However, the effects are usually small and not a substitute for a healthy diet and exercise.

➤ **Long-Term Impact:** The effectiveness for long-term fat loss is limited, and many products lack substantial evidence of sustained benefits.

**Usage:**

➤ **Timing:** Follow product recommendations, typically taking them before workouts or as directed.

> **Considerations:** Be cautious of potential side effects, such as increased heart rate or anxiety, and consult a healthcare provider before starting.

## Understanding When and How to Use Supplements Effectively

1. **Assessing Needs:**

> **Dietary Gaps:** Supplements can be useful for filling gaps in the diet. For example, if you struggle to meet protein needs through food alone, protein powder can help.

> **Specific Goals:** Choose supplements that align with fitness goals, such as creatine for strength or BCAAs for muscle recovery.

2. **Combining with a Balanced Diet:**

> **Supplementation vs. Food:** Supplements should complement, not replace, a balanced diet. Whole foods provide additional nutrients and benefits that supplements alone cannot offer.

3. **Monitoring and Adjusting:**

> **Individual Response:** Track how your body responds to supplements and adjust usage as needed. Not everyone will experience the same benefits.

> **Consult Professionals:** Consider consulting a healthcare provider or nutritionist to ensure

supplements are appropriate for individual health conditions and goals.

## 4.  Avoiding Overuse:

➢ **Dosage Guidelines:** Follow recommended dosages and avoid excessive use, which can lead to adverse effects.

➢ **Quality and Safety:** Choose high-quality supplements from reputable brands to ensure safety and efficacy.

In summary, while supplements can support fitness and health goals, their effectiveness varies based on individual needs and proper usage. Understanding what works and what doesn't, and how to use supplements effectively, can help enhance performance, recovery, and overall well-being.

# Training for Specific Sports

Fitness plans must be tailored to the specific demands of different sports. Each sport has unique requirements that influence the type of training athletes undergo to optimize their performance. This section explores how fitness plans differ for various athletes, including runners, swimmers, basketball players, and bodybuilders, and highlights the role of functional training in enhancing sport-specific performance.

## How Fitness Plans Differ for Athletes

### 1. Runners

**Goals:** Improve endurance, speed, and overall cardiovascular health.

**Training Focus:**

- **Endurance Training:** Long-distance runs and tempo runs to build aerobic capacity and stamina.

- **Speed Work:** Interval training and sprint sessions to enhance speed and running efficiency.

- **Strength Training:** Focus on core strength and lower body exercises such as squats, lunges, and calf raises to support running mechanics and prevent injuries.

➤ **Flexibility:** Regular stretching and mobility work to improve range of motion and reduce the risk of strains.

**Example Routine:**

➤ **Monday:** Long run (60-90 minutes at a moderate pace)

➤ **Tuesday:** Interval training (e.g., 400m sprints with rest intervals)

➤ **Wednesday:** Strength training (e.g., leg presses, hamstring curls)

➤ **Thursday:** Tempo run (20-30 minutes at a challenging pace)

➤ **Friday:** Rest or light cross-training (e.g., cycling)

➤ **Saturday:** Speed work (e.g., 200m sprints)

➤ **Sunday:** Recovery run (30-45 minutes at an easy pace)

## 2.  Swimmers

**Goals:** Enhance swimming technique, build endurance, and improve overall power and flexibility.

**Training Focus:**

➤ **Swimming Drills:** Technique-focused sets to improve stroke efficiency and reduce drag.

➢ **Endurance Training:** Long swim sets and interval training in the pool to build cardiovascular capacity.

➢ **Strength Training:** Focus on upper body strength and core stability, with exercises such as pull-ups, lat pull-downs, and core exercises.

➢ **Dryland Training:** Complementary exercises to enhance power and flexibility, such as resistance bands and plyometric drills.

**Example Routine:**

➢ **Monday:** Technique drills (e.g., 50m sprints focusing on stroke form)

➢ **Tuesday:** Endurance swim (e.g., 2000m continuous swim)

➢ **Wednesday:** Strength training (e.g., bench press, rows)

➢ **Thursday:** Interval training (e.g., 100m sprints with rest)

➢ **Friday:** Flexibility and mobility work (e.g., yoga or stretching)

➢ **Saturday:** Long swim (e.g., 3000m with varied strokes)

➢ **Sunday:** Recovery or light cross-training (e.g., easy jog)

### 3.  Basketball Players

**Goals:** Enhance agility, strength, power, and overall basketball skills.

**Training Focus:**

- **Agility Training:** Drills to improve quickness and reaction time, such as cone drills and ladder exercises.

- **Strength Training:** Focus on lower body strength (e.g., squats, deadlifts) and upper body power (e.g., bench press, shoulder press).

- **Plyometrics:** Jump training and explosive movements to improve vertical leap and quickness.

- **Skill Work:** On-court drills for shooting, dribbling, and defensive skills.

**Example Routine:**

- **Monday:** Strength training (e.g., squats, lunges)

- **Tuesday:** Agility drills (e.g., ladder drills, cone drills)

- **Wednesday:** Skill practice (e.g., shooting, dribbling)

- **Thursday:** Plyometrics (e.g., box jumps, depth jumps)

- **Friday:** Strength training (e.g., bench press, pull-ups)

- ➤ **Saturday:** Scrimmage or game simulation

- ➤ **Sunday:** Rest or active recovery (e.g., light jogging, stretching)

## 4. Bodybuilders

**Goals:** Build muscle mass, increase strength, and improve overall physique aesthetics.

**Training Focus:**

- ➤ **Hypertrophy Training:** High-volume weight training with moderate to heavy weights and multiple sets/reps to induce muscle growth.

- ➤ **Isolation Exercises:** Focus on specific muscle groups to enhance symmetry and definition (e.g., bicep curls, tricep extensions).

- ➤ **Nutrition:** High-protein diet with careful macronutrient balance to support muscle growth and recovery.

- ➤ **Recovery:** Adequate rest and recovery to allow muscle repair and growth.

**Example Routine:**

- ➤ **Monday:** Chest and triceps (e.g., bench press, tricep dips)

- ➤ **Tuesday:** Back and biceps (e.g., pull-ups, bicep curls)

- ➤ **Wednesday:** Legs (e.g., squats, leg presses)

- ➤ **Thursday:** Shoulders and abs (e.g., shoulder press, crunches)

- ➤ **Friday:** Full-body workout or targeted muscle groups

- ➤ **Saturday:** Cardio or active recovery (e.g., light jogging)

- ➤ **Sunday:** Rest

## Functional Training and Its Role in Sport-Specific Performance

**Functional Training:** This type of training focuses on exercises that mimic real-life movements and activities, enhancing the body's ability to perform everyday tasks and specific sports skills.

**Benefits:**

- ➤ **Improved Movement Patterns:** Functional exercises enhance the efficiency and effectiveness of movements relevant to the sport, such as jumping, running, or throwing.

- ➤ **Injury Prevention:** By strengthening muscles and stabilizing joints, functional training can reduce the risk of injuries that might occur during sports activities.

> **Increased Performance:** Functional exercises often involve multiple muscle groups and movement patterns, leading to improvements in overall athletic performance.

**Examples of Functional Training Exercises:**

> **Runners:** Box jumps, lateral shuffles, and resistance band drills to mimic running mechanics and improve explosiveness.

> **Swimmers:** Medicine ball throws, stability ball exercises, and swim cord exercises to enhance power and coordination in the water.

> **Basketball Players:** Agility ladders, plyometric jumps, and rotational exercises to improve quickness, vertical leap, and on-court movement.

> **Bodybuilders:** Functional strength exercises like kettlebell swings and compound movements to enhance muscle coordination and overall strength.

In summary, training for specific sports requires a tailored approach that addresses the unique demands of each sport. By incorporating functional training and focusing on sport-specific skills, athletes can enhance their performance, reduce the risk of injuries, and achieve their fitness goals more effectively.

# Injury Prevention and Recovery

Injury prevention and effective recovery are crucial aspects of maintaining a consistent and successful fitness regimen. Whether you're a seasoned athlete or a fitness enthusiast, understanding best practices for preventing injuries and managing recovery can help you stay on track and achieve your fitness goals.

## Best Practices for Preventing Injuries

### 1. Proper Warm-Up and Cool-Down

**Warm-Up:** Preparing your body for exercise is essential to reduce the risk of injury. A good warm-up increases blood flow to the muscles, enhances flexibility, and primes the body for more intense physical activity.

**Warm-Up Tips:**

- **Dynamic Stretches:** Incorporate movements that mimic the activity you're about to perform, such as leg swings, arm circles, and high knees.

- **Gradual Intensity:** Start with low-intensity activities and gradually increase the intensity to prepare your muscles and joints.

**Cool-Down:** Cooling down after exercise helps to gradually lower your heart rate and relax your muscles, reducing the risk of soreness and stiffness.

## Cool-Down Tips:

- ➢ **Static Stretches:** Perform static stretches focusing on the major muscle groups used during your workout. Hold each stretch for 20-30 seconds.

- ➢ **Breathing Exercises:** Practice deep breathing to help your body transition back to a resting state.

## 2. Proper Technique and Form

**Importance of Technique:** Using correct form during exercises is crucial for avoiding injuries and ensuring that you're targeting the intended muscle groups effectively.

## Technique Tips:

- ➢ **Learn Proper Form:** Seek guidance from a certified trainer or use instructional resources to learn the correct technique for each exercise.

- ➢ **Use Proper Equipment:** Ensure that equipment is adjusted to your body size and strength level, and use supportive footwear when necessary.

## 3. Gradual Progression

**Avoiding the Overload:** Progress gradually to avoid overloading your muscles and joints, which can lead to strain and injury.

## Progression Tips:

- ➤ **Increase Intensity Gradually:** Increase weights, repetitions, or duration of exercise in small increments.

- ➤ **Listen to Your Body:** Pay attention to signs of fatigue or discomfort, and adjust your training intensity as needed.

## 4. Cross-Training and Variety

**Benefits of Cross-Training:** Incorporating a variety of exercises into your routine can help prevent overuse injuries and improve overall fitness.

## Cross-Training Tips:

- ➤ **Mix It Up:** Alternate between different types of exercises, such as cardio, strength training, and flexibility work.

- ➤ **Rest Days:** Schedule regular rest days to allow your body to recover and prevent overuse injuries.

## 5. Strengthening Supporting Muscles

**Importance of Support:** Strengthening the muscles that support your primary muscle groups can help prevent injuries and improve overall stability.

## Supporting Muscle Tips:

- ➤ **Core Strength:** Focus on exercises that strengthen your core muscles, such as planks and abdominal exercises.

➤ **Joint Stability:** Include exercises that enhance joint stability, such as stability ball exercises and resistance band drills.

127

# How to Recover Quickly and Safely from Injuries

## 1. Immediate First Aid

**R.I.C.E. Method:** The R.I.C.E. method is a standard approach for managing acute injuries, such as sprains and strains.

**R.I.C.E. Components:**

- **Rest:** Avoid activities that cause pain or discomfort.

- **Ice:** Apply ice to the injured area to reduce swelling and inflammation. Use an ice pack for 15-20 minutes at a time.

- **Compression:** Use an elastic bandage to compress the injured area and reduce swelling.

- **Elevation:** Keep the injured area elevated above heart level to minimize swelling.

## 2. Consult a Healthcare Professional

**When to Seek Help:** For severe injuries or if you experience persistent pain, swelling, or limited movement, consult a healthcare professional for a proper diagnosis and treatment plan.

## Consultation Tips:

- **Describe Symptoms:** Provide a detailed account of your symptoms and how the injury occurred.

- **Follow Recommendations:** Adhere to the treatment plan and rehabilitation exercises prescribed by your healthcare provider.

## 3. Gradual Return to Activity

**Rehabilitation:** Gradually reintroduce physical activity as you recover to avoid re-injury and build strength in the affected area.

## Return-to-Activity Tips:

- **Follow a Rehabilitation Program:** Engage in a structured rehabilitation program to regain strength and flexibility.

- **Start Slowly:** Begin with low-intensity activities and gradually increase intensity as your injury heals.

## 4. Nutrition and Hydration

**Supporting Recovery:** Proper nutrition and hydration play a significant role in the healing process and overall recovery.

## Nutrition Tips:

- **Balanced Diet:** Consume a balanced diet rich in proteins, vitamins, and minerals to support tissue repair and reduce inflammation.

> **Hydration:** Stay well-hydrated to aid in recovery and maintain joint lubrication.

## 5. Mental and Emotional Support

**Psychological Aspects:** Injury recovery can be challenging both physically and emotionally. Seek support to stay positive and motivated during your rehabilitation process.

**Support Tips:**

> **Set Realistic Goals:** Set small, achievable goals to track progress and stay motivated.

> **Seek Support:** Engage in conversations with friends, family, or a counselor to address any emotional challenges related to your injury.

## 6. Long-Term Prevention

**Preventing Future Injuries:** Implement strategies to prevent future injuries by addressing any underlying issues and maintaining a well-rounded fitness routine.

**Prevention Tips:**

> **Regular Check-Ups:** Schedule periodic assessments with a healthcare professional or trainer to address any potential issues.

> **Ongoing Education:** Stay informed about best practices for injury prevention and recovery to continually improve your fitness regimen.

In summary, injury prevention and recovery require a multifaceted approach that includes proper warm-up, correct technique, gradual progression, and effective recovery strategies. By following these best practices and seeking appropriate support, you can minimize the risk of injuries and ensure a safe and successful fitness journey.

# The Role of Genetics in Fitness

Genetics play a significant role in determining various aspects of fitness, including body type, metabolism, and athletic potential. Understanding how your genetic makeup influences these factors can help you tailor your fitness plan more effectively to suit your individual needs and optimize your performance.

## How Your Genetics Influence Body Type, Metabolism, and Athletic Potential

### 1. Body Type

**Genetic Influence on Body Type:** Your genetic blueprint largely dictates your body type, which can be categorized into three primary types: ectomorph, mesomorph, and endomorph. Each body type has distinct characteristics that can affect how you gain muscle, lose fat, and respond to different types of exercise.

**Body Type Descriptions:**

➤ **Ectomorph:** Individuals with an ectomorph body type are typically lean with a smaller frame, narrow shoulders, and low body fat. They often find it challenging to gain weight or build muscle mass.

This body type may benefit from a fitness plan focused on strength training with an emphasis on calorie-dense nutrition to support muscle growth.

➤ **Mesomorph:** Mesomorphs have a more muscular and athletic build with broad shoulders, a narrower waist, and an easier time gaining muscle and strength. They are often naturally strong and respond well to a balanced fitness regimen that includes both resistance training and cardiovascular exercises.

➤ **Endomorph:** Endomorphs generally have a rounder body shape with a higher percentage of body fat and a tendency to gain weight easily. A fitness plan for this body type might focus on a combination of resistance training and high-intensity interval training (HIIT) to manage body fat and improve overall fitness.

## 2. Metabolism

**Genetic Influence on Metabolism:** Your metabolism—the process by which your body converts food into energy—is influenced by your genes. Genetic variations can affect how efficiently your body burns calories, stores fat, and processes nutrients.

**Metabolic Variations:**

➤ **Basal Metabolic Rate (BMR):** Genetics can influence your BMR, which is the number of calories your body needs to maintain basic physiological functions at rest. Individuals with a higher BMR burn more calories at rest, while those with a lower BMR may need to be more mindful of their caloric intake.

➤ **Fat Storage and Utilization:** Some people have a genetic predisposition to store fat more readily or utilize fat for energy differently. For example, variations in genes related to fat metabolism can influence how your body stores or burns fat, affecting your overall body composition and weight management efforts.

## 3. Athletic Potential

**Genetic Influence on Athletic Performance:** Genetics also play a role in determining your potential for various athletic activities. Factors such as muscle fiber composition, cardiovascular efficiency, and response to training can be influenced by your genetic makeup.

**Genetic Factors Affecting Athletic Performance:**

➤ **Muscle Fiber Types:** There are two main types of muscle fibers—fast-twitch and slow-twitch. Fast-twitch fibers are responsible for explosive, high-intensity activities like sprinting, while slow-twitch fibers are more suited for endurance activities like long-distance running. Your proportion of these fibers is largely genetic and can impact your performance in different sports.

> **Cardiovascular Efficiency:** Genetics can influence your cardiovascular system's efficiency, affecting how well your heart and lungs perform during aerobic activities. Some individuals may have a natural advantage in endurance sports due to their genetic predisposition for better cardiovascular function.

> **Response to Training:** Genetic variations can affect how your body responds to different types of training. Some people may experience rapid gains in strength and muscle mass with resistance training, while others may need more time to see significant results. Understanding your genetic response to training can help you optimize your fitness plan.

## How to Adapt Your Fitness Plan Based on Genetic Predispositions

### 1. Tailoring Your Workouts

**Customized Training Programs:** Adapt your fitness plan to align with your body type, metabolic rate, and athletic potential. This personalized approach ensures that you're engaging in exercises that complement your genetic strengths and address areas where you may need additional support.

**Adaptation Tips:**

> **Body Type Considerations:** Choose exercises that align with your body type. For example, ectomorphs

may benefit from resistance training with heavy weights to build muscle, while endomorphs may focus on a combination of strength training and cardiovascular workouts to manage body fat.

➤ **Metabolism Management:** Adjust your caloric intake and macronutrient distribution based on your metabolic rate. Individuals with a higher BMR may need to consume more calories to support their energy needs, while those with a lower BMR may need to monitor their intake more closely.

➤ **Athletic Focus:** Design your workout program based on your genetic strengths. If you have a higher proportion of fast-twitch muscle fibers, you might excel in high-intensity activities and should focus on explosive exercises. Conversely, if you have more slow-twitch fibers, endurance training could be more beneficial.

## 2. Nutritional Adjustments

**Genetic-Based Nutrition:** Adapt your diet to support your fitness goals and genetic predispositions. Understanding how your body metabolizes different nutrients can help you make more informed choices about your diet.

**Nutritional Adjustments Tips:**

➤ **Macronutrient Ratios:** Adjust your macronutrient ratios (protein, carbohydrates, and fats) based on your metabolic needs. For example, individuals with a higher BMR may require more protein and carbohydrates to support muscle growth and recovery.

> **Nutrient Timing:** Consider the timing of your meals and snacks to optimize performance and recovery. Eating a balanced meal or snack before and after workouts can help improve energy levels and enhance recovery.

## 3. Monitoring and Adjusting

**Ongoing Assessment:** Regularly assess your progress and make adjustments to your fitness plan based on your results and any changes in your genetic factors.

**Monitoring Tips:**

> **Track Progress:** Keep track of your performance, body composition, and overall fitness to determine if your current plan is effective. Use metrics such as strength gains, endurance improvements, and changes in body measurements to evaluate your progress.

> **Adjust as Needed:** Be prepared to make adjustments to your fitness plan based on your results and any new insights into your genetic predispositions. Continuously refine your approach to ensure that

you're optimizing your performance and achieving your goals.

In summary, understanding the role of genetics in fitness can provide valuable insights into how your body responds to different types of exercise, nutrition, and training. By tailoring your fitness plan to your genetic predispositions, you can enhance your performance, achieve better results, and ultimately reach your fitness goals more effectively.

# Importance of Mobility and Flexibility

**Mobility** and **flexibility** are often used interchangeably, but they refer to different aspects of physical function. While flexibility relates to the range of motion in a specific joint or muscle, mobility encompasses the ability to move freely and comfortably through a full range of motion without restrictions or discomfort. Both are crucial for optimizing workout performance and maintaining long-term health.

## How Mobility and Flexibility Affect Workout Performance and Long-Term Health

### 1. Impact on Workout Performance

**Injury Prevention:** Adequate mobility and flexibility are essential for injury prevention. Tight muscles or restricted joints can lead to compensatory movements that increase the risk of strain or injury. For example, limited hip mobility can result in poor squat form, putting extra stress on the lower back. By improving flexibility and mobility, you reduce the risk of injuries related to improper movement patterns.

**Enhanced Range of Motion:** Improved flexibility and mobility allow for a greater range of motion in exercises. This enables you to perform movements more effectively and achieve better muscle activation.

For instance, greater shoulder flexibility enhances your ability to perform exercises like overhead presses and pull-ups with proper form, leading to more effective workouts and better results.

**Better Performance in Functional Movements:** Mobility and flexibility contribute to functional movement patterns, which are essential for both athletic performance and daily activities. Activities such as running, jumping, and lifting require a full range of motion and proper joint function. Improved mobility helps in executing these movements efficiently and with reduced risk of injury.

## 2. Impact on Long-Term Health

**Joint Health:** Maintaining good mobility and flexibility helps keep your joints healthy by promoting smooth and efficient movement. Regular stretching and mobility exercises can prevent stiffness and joint degeneration, reducing the risk of conditions such as osteoarthritis.

**Posture Improvement:** Poor flexibility and mobility can contribute to postural imbalances, leading to back pain and other musculoskeletal issues. Stretching and mobility exercises help to correct imbalances, improve posture, and alleviate discomfort associated with poor alignment.

**Increased Quality of Life:** Flexibility and mobility are crucial for maintaining an active and independent lifestyle as you age. Being able to move freely and without pain enhances overall quality of life and reduces the likelihood of developing physical limitations.

## Exercises and Routines to Improve Mobility and Flexibility

### 1. Stretching Exercises

**Static Stretching:** This involves holding a stretch for a prolonged period (15-60 seconds) to lengthen the muscles and improve flexibility. It is typically performed after a workout to aid in muscle recovery and maintain flexibility.

**Examples:**

- **Hamstring Stretch:** Sit on the ground with one leg extended and the other leg bent. Reach toward the toes of the extended leg while keeping your back straight.

- **Quadriceps Stretch:** Stand on one leg and pull the opposite heel toward your glutes. Hold onto your ankle with your hand and keep your knees close together.

**Dynamic Stretching:** This involves moving parts of your body through their full range of motion in a controlled manner. Dynamic stretches are often used as part of a warm-up routine to prepare the muscles and joints for exercise.

**Examples:**

➤ **Leg Swings:** Stand on one leg and swing the other leg forward and backward in a controlled manner. This helps to loosen up the hip joint.

➤ **Arm Circles:** Extend your arms out to the sides and make small circles, gradually increasing the size of the circles. This warms up the shoulder joints.

### 2.  Mobility Exercises

**Joint Mobility Drills:** These exercises target the range of motion of specific joints and help to improve joint function. They can be incorporated into your warm-up routine or performed independently.

**Examples:**

➤ **Hip Circles:** Stand with your feet shoulder-width apart and move your hips in circular motions. This exercise enhances hip joint mobility.

➤ **Thoracic Rotations:** Sit or stand with a straight back and place one hand behind your head. Rotate your torso to one side, then return to the starting position. This improves thoracic spine mobility.

**Foam Rolling:** Foam rolling is a form of self-myofascial release that helps to release muscle tightness and improve mobility. It involves using a foam roller to apply pressure to different muscle groups, aiding in muscle recovery and flexibility.

**Examples:**

- **Quadriceps Foam Roll:** Lie face down and place a foam roller under your thighs. Roll back and forth slowly to target the quadriceps muscles.

- **Calf Foam Roll:** Sit on the ground with your legs extended and place a foam roller under your calves. Roll from the back of your knees to your ankles.

### 3. Yoga and Pilates

**Yoga:** Yoga combines stretching, strength, and balance to improve overall flexibility and mobility. It involves a series of poses that target different muscle groups and joints, promoting relaxation and flexibility.

**Examples:**

- **Downward Dog:** Start on your hands and knees, then lift your hips toward the ceiling, straightening your legs and arms. This pose stretches the hamstrings, calves, and shoulders.

- **Cat-Cow Stretch:** Begin on all fours, alternate between arching your back (cat pose) and dipping it (cow pose). This sequence improves spinal flexibility and mobility.

**Pilates:** Pilates focuses on core strength, stability, and flexibility. It involves controlled movements and exercises that enhance posture, balance, and overall flexibility.

**Examples:**

➤ **The Hundred:** Lie on your back with your legs lifted and bent at a 90-degree angle. Pump your arms up and down while engaging your core. This exercise improves core strength and flexibility.

➤ **Spine Stretch:** Sit with your legs extended and reach forward to touch your toes while keeping your back straight. This stretch targets the spine and hamstrings.

## Conclusion

Mobility and flexibility are fundamental components of an effective fitness regimen and contribute significantly to long-term health and well-being. By incorporating a variety of stretching and mobility exercises, foam rolling, and practices like yoga and Pilates, you can enhance your workout performance, prevent injuries, and maintain optimal physical function throughout your life. Prioritizing these aspects of fitness ensures a well-rounded approach to achieving your fitness goals and supporting your overall health.

# Building Sustainable Fitness Habits

Creating and maintaining sustainable fitness habits is essential for achieving long-term health and wellness goals. Unlike quick fixes or fad diets, sustainable habits focus on integrating fitness into your lifestyle in a way that is both manageable and enjoyable. Here's how you can build and maintain these habits:

## How to Stay Consistent with Workouts and Nutrition Over the Long Term

### 1. Set Realistic Goals

**Define Clear, Achievable Objectives:** Setting specific, measurable, and realistic goals helps provide direction and motivation. Instead of vague goals like "get fit," opt for concrete targets such as "complete a 30-minute workout three times a week" or "incorporate a serving of vegetables into every meal."

**Break Goals into Smaller Milestones:** Large goals can be overwhelming. Breaking them down into smaller, manageable milestones makes them more achievable. Celebrate these small victories to stay motivated and on track.

## 2.  Create a Structured Plan

**Develop a Routine:** Establishing a consistent workout schedule and meal plan is crucial. Allocate specific times for exercise and meal preparation to make these activities a regular part of your day.

**Plan Workouts and Meals Ahead:** Planning ahead helps to avoid last-minute excuses and ensures that you stay prepared. Use a fitness app or planner to schedule workouts and grocery lists to simplify meal prep.

## 3.  Find Activities You Enjoy

**Choose Exercises You Like:** Enjoyable workouts are easier to stick with. Experiment with different types of exercises—such as swimming, cycling, or dancing—to find what you enjoy the most.

**Incorporate Variety:** Mixing up your workouts can prevent boredom and keep you engaged. Try different activities or adjust the intensity to keep things interesting.

## 4.  Make Nutrition Simple and Accessible

**Prepare Meals in Advance:** Meal prepping saves time and reduces the temptation to make unhealthy choices. Prepare and portion meals for the week to ensure you have healthy options readily available.

**Keep Healthy Snacks on Hand:** Stock up on nutritious snacks like fruits, nuts, and yogurt to avoid reaching for junk food when you're hungry.

**5. Track Progress and Stay Accountable**

**Use a Journal or App:** Tracking your workouts, nutrition, and progress helps maintain motivation and provides insight into your habits. Apps like MyFitnessPal or Fitbit can assist in monitoring your goals.

**Seek Support:** Share your goals with friends, family, or a workout buddy. Having a support system keeps you accountable and can provide encouragement during challenging times.

## Strategies to Break Through Motivation Slumps and Plateaus

**1. Reassess and Adjust Goals**

**Evaluate Your Progress:** Regularly review your goals and progress. If you're experiencing a plateau, reassess your objectives and make adjustments to your routine or goals.

**Set New Challenges:** Introducing new challenges or goals can reignite motivation. This could involve increasing your workout intensity, trying a new sport, or setting a new personal record.

## 2.  Change Up Your Routine

**Try New Workouts:** A change in your workout routine can help break through plateaus and keep things exciting. Experiment with new exercises, fitness classes, or training methods.

**Incorporate Different Modalities:** Adding variety to your routine, such as combining strength training with cardio or incorporating flexibility exercises like yoga, can help maintain interest and address different aspects of fitness.

## 3.  Focus on the Positive

**Celebrate Small Wins:** Acknowledge and celebrate your achievements, no matter how small. Recognizing your progress can boost motivation and remind you of how far you've come.

**Practice Self-Compassion:** It's normal to experience ups and downs in your fitness journey. Be kind to yourself during setbacks and use them as learning opportunities rather than reasons to give up.

## 4.  Reconnect with Your "Why"

**Reflect on Your Motivation:** Revisit the reasons why you started your fitness journey. Whether it's improving health, feeling more energetic, or achieving a personal goal, reconnecting with your underlying motivation can help reignite your drive.

**Visualize Success:** Visualization techniques can enhance motivation. Imagine yourself reaching your goals and the positive outcomes associated with your efforts.

## 5.  Seek Professional Guidance

**Consult a Trainer or Nutritionist:** A fitness professional can provide personalized advice and help you overcome plateaus. They can design a tailored workout plan or adjust your nutrition strategy to keep you progressing.

**Join a Fitness Group or Class:** Group settings provide social support and structured routines. Participating in group workouts or classes can offer a sense of community and motivation.

## Conclusion

Building and maintaining sustainable fitness habits requires a combination of realistic goal-setting, structured planning, enjoyable activities, and effective tracking. By focusing on consistency, adapting to challenges, and staying motivated, you can create lasting habits that contribute to long-term health and fitness success. Remember that fitness is a lifelong journey, and the key is to make it a manageable and enjoyable part of your daily life

# Myths and Misconceptions in Fitness

Fitness is a field where misinformation can easily spread, leading many to adopt ineffective or even harmful practices. Understanding the truth behind common fitness myths is essential for achieving your goals efficiently and safely. Below, we debunk several prevalent myths and clarify the facts, providing detailed explanations and examples to illustrate the points.

## Debunking Common Fitness Myths

### 1. Spot Reduction:

**The Myth:** Spot reduction is the belief that you can target fat loss in specific areas of your body by performing exercises that focus on those areas. For instance, many people do countless abdominal exercises like crunches and sit-ups with the expectation that this will lead to a flat stomach and reduced belly fat.

**The Reality:** Spot reduction is a misconception. Research shows that you cannot control where your body loses fat. Fat loss occurs through overall body fat reduction, not from localized exercise. When you perform exercises for a specific muscle group, you are strengthening and building that muscle, but fat loss comes from a combination of overall calorie deficit and genetics.

**Example:** Imagine you are doing 100 sit-ups a day, hoping this will reduce your belly fat. While these sit-ups will strengthen your abdominal muscles, they won't necessarily reduce the fat covering those muscles. Instead, incorporating a well-rounded fitness routine that includes cardiovascular exercise (like running or cycling), strength training, and a balanced diet will help reduce overall body fat, including in the abdominal area.

## 2. Fasting for Weight Loss:

**The Myth:** Fasting, including methods like intermittent fasting, is often touted as a quick way to lose weight by enhancing fat burning. Some believe that not eating for certain periods forces the body to burn fat more efficiently.

**The Reality:** While intermittent fasting can be effective for some individuals, it is not a universal solution for weight loss. Weight loss fundamentally depends on creating a calorie deficit—burning more calories than you consume. Fasting might help some people manage their calorie intake but isn't inherently better than other methods of calorie control.

**Example:** Consider a person who fasts for 16 hours a day but compensates by eating large amounts of high-calorie foods during the remaining 8 hours. This approach might not lead to weight loss if the overall calorie intake exceeds the calories burned. Instead, focusing on a balanced diet and regular exercise is a more sustainable approach for long-term weight management.

## 3. Fat-Burning Zones:

**The Myth:** The concept of fat-burning zones suggests that exercising at a lower intensity keeps you in a zone where your body supposedly burns a higher percentage of calories from fat compared to higher-intensity exercise.

**The Reality:** While it is true that lower-intensity exercise burns a higher percentage of calories from fat, higher-intensity exercise burns more total calories, including fat. The most effective way to burn fat is to focus on overall calorie expenditure, which can be achieved through both high and low-intensity workouts.

**Example:** Running at a moderate pace (70% of your maximum heart rate) burns a higher percentage of fat calories, but running at a high intensity (85% of your maximum heart rate) burns more total calories, including fat. Incorporating both high and low-intensity workouts can be more effective for overall fat loss.

## 4. More Exercise Equals Better Results:

**The Myth:** There is a belief that spending more time exercising will lead to better results. This often leads to overtraining, where individuals work out excessively in the hope of achieving faster progress.

**The Reality:** Quality and consistency of exercise are more important than quantity. Overtraining can lead to injuries, fatigue, and decreased performance. A well-balanced exercise program that includes adequate rest and recovery will provide better results than excessive training.

**Example:** Imagine someone who exercises intensely for 2 hours daily without proper rest. They might experience burnout or injuries, which can hinder progress. In contrast, a balanced routine with moderate intensity, proper rest, and recovery days will lead to more sustainable improvements in fitness and health.

## 5. Supplements Are a Quick Fix:

**The Myth:** Many believe that supplements can quickly solve fitness problems or replace a poor diet. Supplements like protein powders, creatine, and fat burners are often advertised as quick fixes.

**The Reality:** Supplements can support a well-rounded fitness regimen but are not a substitute for a healthy diet and regular exercise. The most significant benefits come from a balanced diet rich in whole foods and consistent exercise.

**Example:** A person taking protein supplements may believe they can skip consuming protein-rich foods like chicken or legumes. However, a well-rounded diet that includes natural food sources of protein, combined with targeted supplementation if necessary, will provide better results for muscle building and recovery.

# Nutrition and Diet

# Functional vs. Aesthetic Fitness

In the realm of fitness, there are two primary goals that individuals often pursue: functional fitness and aesthetic fitness. Both approaches have their unique benefits and contribute to overall well-being, but understanding the differences and how to balance them is essential for a comprehensive fitness regimen. Here's a detailed comparison:

## Difference Between Training for Functionality vs. Appearance

### 1. Functional Fitness:

**Definition:** Functional fitness focuses on exercises that enhance your ability to perform everyday activities. It emphasizes practical movements that improve strength, balance, coordination, and flexibility. The goal is to train your body to handle real-life tasks more effectively and reduce the risk of injury.

**Key Characteristics:**

- **Movement Patterns:** Exercises often replicate natural movement patterns such as squatting, lifting, bending, and twisting.

- **Core Stability:** Emphasizes strengthening the core to support overall body stability and functional performance.

- **Versatility:** Incorporates a variety of exercises that improve multiple aspects of physical fitness, such as agility, endurance, and flexibility.

**Examples:**

- **Squats:** Mimic the action of sitting down and standing up, which aids in everyday activities like getting up from a chair or picking up objects from the floor.

- **Lunges:** Improve balance and coordination, which are beneficial for walking, climbing stairs, and navigating uneven surfaces.

- **Kettlebell Swings:** Enhance hip strength, core stability, and cardiovascular endurance, which can improve overall functional capacity.

## 2. Aesthetic Fitness:

**Definition:** Aesthetic fitness is centered around achieving a specific physical appearance, often characterized by muscle definition and low body fat. It focuses on bodybuilding and sculpting the body to achieve a particular look, such as increased muscle size and a toned physique.

## Key Characteristics:

➤ **Muscle Isolation:** Exercises often target specific muscle groups to enhance their size and definition.

➤ **Body Composition:** Aims to reduce body fat while increasing muscle mass to achieve a more defined and sculpted appearance.

➤ **Visual Goals:** The primary objective is to improve physical appearance rather than functional capacity.

## Examples:

➤ **Bodybuilding Workouts:** Include exercises like bicep curls, tricep extensions, and chest presses to isolate and build individual muscles for a more defined physique.

➤ **Isolation Exercises:** Focus on specific muscles, such as calf raises for the calves or leg extensions for the quadriceps, to enhance muscle definition and appearance.

➤ **High-Volume Training:** Involves performing multiple sets and reps to achieve muscle hypertrophy and improve visual aesthetics.

## Why Balancing Both is Crucial for a Well-Rounded Physique

Balancing functional and aesthetic fitness is essential for several reasons:

1. **Comprehensive Health Benefits:**

- ➤ **Functional Fitness:** Improves your ability to perform daily tasks, enhances overall physical capabilities, and reduces the risk of injuries. It ensures that you have the strength, coordination, and flexibility to handle real-life activities effectively.

- ➤ **Aesthetic Fitness:** Contributes to a well-defined physique, which can boost confidence and improve body image. It helps in building muscle size and achieving a toned appearance.

2. **Injury Prevention and Performance:**

- ➤ **Functional Training:** Strengthens stabilizing muscles and improves joint mobility, which can prevent injuries and enhance performance in various physical activities. It also supports proper movement patterns and overall body mechanics.

- ➤ **Aesthetic Training:** While it focuses on muscle growth and appearance, it can also contribute to strength gains that support functional performance. However, overemphasis on aesthetics without functional training can lead to muscle imbalances and increased risk of injury.

## 3. Motivation and Adherence:

➤ **Variety in Training:** Combining functional and aesthetic training keeps your workouts diverse and engaging. It prevents monotony and helps maintain motivation by addressing both performance and appearance goals.

➤ **Holistic Approach:** Balancing both approaches ensures that you achieve a well-rounded fitness regimen that not only improves your physical appearance but also enhances your functional abilities and overall health.

## 4. Long-Term Sustainability:

➤ **Functional Fitness:** Ensures that you build a solid foundation of physical capabilities that support long-term health and performance. It prepares you for various activities and challenges, contributing to overall well-being.

➤ **Aesthetic Fitness:** Provides visual goals and satisfaction, which can be motivating and rewarding. However, focusing solely on aesthetics without considering functionality may lead to imbalances and limitations in physical performance.

## Example of Balancing Both Approaches

**Scenario:** Imagine a fitness enthusiast who trains solely for aesthetics by performing isolation exercises and focusing on muscle growth. While they achieve a well-defined physique, they may struggle with functional tasks such as lifting heavy objects or maintaining balance during everyday activities.

To address this, the individual incorporates functional training into their routine. They add exercises like squats, lunges, and kettlebell swings, which improve overall strength, stability, and mobility. This balanced approach enhances their functional capabilities while maintaining their aesthetic goals.

## Conclusion:

Balancing functional and aesthetic fitness is crucial for achieving a well-rounded physique and overall health. By integrating both approaches into your fitness routine, you can enhance your physical appearance, improve functional performance, and support long-term well-being. A comprehensive fitness regimen that addresses both functionality and aesthetics ensures that you achieve your goals effectively and sustainably.

# The Role of a Fitness Coach

**How a Coach Can Tailor Programs to Individual Needs**

A fitness coach plays a crucial role in designing and implementing exercise programs that are tailored specifically to each individual's needs, goals, and limitations. This personalized approach is essential for achieving optimal results and minimizing the risk of injury.

1. **Assessing Individual Needs:** The first step in tailoring a program involves a thorough assessment of the client's current fitness level, health status, and personal goals. For example, if a client's goal is to lose weight and improve cardiovascular health, the coach might start with an initial fitness test to evaluate endurance, strength, and flexibility. This assessment helps the coach understand where the client stands and what specific areas need attention.

2. **Setting Personalized Goals:** Once the assessment is complete, the coach collaborates with the client to set realistic and achievable goals. These goals could range from losing a specific amount of weight, building muscle, or improving overall

endurance. For instance, if a client is aiming to run a marathon, the coach will design a training plan that gradually increases mileage while incorporating rest days and cross-training to prevent overuse injuries.

3. **Designing Customized Workout Plans:** Based on the assessment and goals, the coach creates a workout plan that is tailored to the client's needs. This plan includes a mix of exercises that target different fitness components, such as strength, endurance, flexibility, and balance. For example, a client with joint issues might receive a program focused on low-impact exercises like swimming or cycling, while someone looking to build muscle might have a plan centered around resistance training.

4. **Monitoring Progress and Adjusting the Plan:** A fitness coach continually monitors the client's progress through regular check-ins and assessments. This allows the coach to make necessary adjustments to the program based on the client's feedback and progress. For instance, if a client is not seeing the expected results or is experiencing discomfort, the coach can modify the exercises, adjust the intensity, or change the approach to better align with the client's evolving needs.

5.  **Providing Education and Guidance:** In addition to designing workout plans, a coach educates clients about proper exercise techniques, nutrition, and lifestyle habits. This knowledge empowers clients to make informed decisions about their fitness journey. For example, a coach might teach a client proper form for squats to ensure they perform the exercise safely and effectively, thereby reducing the risk of injury and maximizing the benefits.

By tailoring programs to individual needs, a fitness coach ensures that each client receives a personalized approach that addresses their specific goals and challenges. This customized support enhances the likelihood of success and helps clients achieve their fitness objectives in a safe and efficient manner.

# Finding the Right Coach

## What Qualifications and Qualities to Look For

Choosing the right fitness coach can significantly impact your journey towards achieving your fitness goals. Here are key qualifications and qualities to consider when selecting a coach:

1. **Relevant Certifications:** A qualified fitness coach should hold certifications from reputable organizations that demonstrate their knowledge and expertise. Look for certifications from well-regarded institutions such as the American College of Sports Medicine (ACSM), National Academy of Sports Medicine (NASM), or International Sports Sciences Association (ISSA). These certifications ensure that the coach has undergone rigorous training and is knowledgeable about exercise science, nutrition, and safe practices.

2. **Experience and Specialization:** Consider the coach's experience and whether their specialization aligns with your fitness goals. For example, if you're aiming for muscle building and strength training, a coach with a background in bodybuilding or strength conditioning might be more suitable. If you're recovering from an injury,

a coach with experience in injury rehabilitation and corrective exercise would be beneficial. Look for a coach who has a track record of successfully working with clients who have similar goals or challenges to yours.

3. **Education and Knowledge:** In addition to certifications, a coach's educational background can provide insight into their expertise. Coaches with degrees in fields such as exercise physiology, sports science, or nutrition often bring a deeper understanding of the body and its functions. This knowledge allows them to create more effective and scientifically grounded training programs.

4. **Communication Skills:** Effective communication is crucial for a successful coaching relationship. A good coach should be able to clearly explain exercise techniques, provide constructive feedback, and listen to your concerns. They should also be approachable and willing to answer questions, ensuring that you feel comfortable and confident in your training.

5. **Motivation and Support:** Look for a coach who demonstrates enthusiasm and motivation. They should be able to inspire and encourage you, helping you stay focused and committed to your goals. A coach who offers emotional support and understands the psychological aspects of fitness

can be particularly valuable in maintaining motivation and overcoming challenges.

6. **Professionalism and Integrity:** A coach should exhibit professionalism in their conduct, including punctuality, respect, and adherence to ethical standards. They should provide honest assessments and set realistic expectations, avoiding false promises or unrealistic claims about quick results.

## How to Evaluate if a Coach is a Good Fit for You

Finding a coach who is the right fit for you involves evaluating several factors beyond just qualifications:

1. **Initial Consultation:** Many coaches offer a free initial consultation or assessment. Use this opportunity to discuss your fitness goals, ask questions about their approach, and gauge their response. Pay attention to how well they understand your needs and whether their proposed plan aligns with your expectations.

2. **Compatibility and Rapport:** Assess whether you feel comfortable and compatible with the coach. A good working relationship is essential for long-term success. During the consultation, observe their communication style and how they interact with you. A positive and respectful rapport

can enhance the effectiveness of the coaching relationship.

3. **Client Reviews and Testimonials:** Seek feedback from current or past clients. Reviews and testimonials can provide insight into the coach's effectiveness and their ability to deliver results. Look for testimonials that highlight the coach's strengths in areas relevant to your goals, such as client satisfaction, progress, and overall experience.

4. **Trial Sessions:** Consider starting with a few trial sessions to experience the coach's training style and approach. This allows you to assess how well their methods align with your preferences and whether their coaching style motivates and supports you effectively.

5. **Flexibility and Adaptability:** Evaluate the coach's willingness to adapt their methods based on your feedback and progress. A good coach should be open to adjusting the program as needed to address any concerns or changes in your fitness journey.

6. **Cost and Logistics:** Consider the cost of coaching and whether it fits within your budget. Additionally, assess the logistics such as location, session times, and availability. Ensuring that these practical

aspects align with your schedule and preferences is important for maintaining consistency in your training.

By carefully considering these factors, you can find a fitness coach who not only possesses the necessary qualifications and expertise but also aligns with your personal goals and needs. A well-matched coach can make a significant difference in your fitness journey, providing the guidance, support, and motivation necessary to achieve your desired outcomes.

# The Impact of Coaching on Motivation and Accountability

## How a Coach Can Help You Stay Motivated

1. **Personalized Goal Setting:** A fitness coach plays a crucial role in setting realistic and personalized goals that align with your aspirations and current fitness level. By breaking down larger goals into smaller, achievable milestones, a coach helps you stay focused and motivated. For instance, if your primary goal is to lose 20 pounds, a coach might set monthly targets such as losing 2 pounds each month. This incremental approach keeps you motivated as you experience regular progress and celebrate small victories along the way.

2. **Customized Workouts:** A coach designs tailored workout programs that match your individual needs, preferences, and fitness levels. This personalization not only enhances the effectiveness of your training but also keeps you engaged. For example, if you enjoy high-intensity interval training (HIIT) but find weightlifting tedious, a coach might incorporate HIIT into your routine while gradually introducing weightlifting exercises in a way that feels manageable and interesting.

3. **Regular Progress Tracking:** Tracking progress is a powerful motivator, and a coach provides regular assessments to measure your achievements. By monitoring key metrics such as weight, strength, endurance, or flexibility, a coach helps you visualize your progress and stay motivated. This ongoing feedback allows you to see the tangible results of your efforts and reinforces your commitment to your fitness goals.

4. **Encouragement and Support:** A coach offers consistent encouragement and emotional support throughout your fitness journey. They celebrate your successes, provide constructive feedback, and help you overcome obstacles. For instance, if you hit a plateau or face a challenging period, your coach's support and reassurance can boost your morale and keep you motivated to push through difficult times.

5. **Structured Routine and Accountability:** Having scheduled sessions with a coach creates a structured routine and ensures accountability. Knowing that you have an appointment with your coach can motivate you to adhere to your workout plan and make healthier choices. This regular commitment helps maintain consistency, which is essential for long-term success. For example, if you have a session planned for three times a week, you're

more likely to stay committed to your training schedule compared to a self-guided plan without set appointments.

6. **Education and Inspiration:** A coach educates you about fitness principles, nutrition, and effective training techniques. This knowledge not only empowers you to make informed decisions but also inspires you to continue your fitness journey. For instance, learning about the benefits of strength training or understanding how proper nutrition supports recovery can motivate you to incorporate these practices into your routine.

## Strategies for Effective Communication with Your Coach

1. **Open and Honest Dialogue:** Effective communication begins with openness and honesty. Clearly express your goals, preferences, and any concerns you may have. If you have specific fitness goals, share them with your coach so they can tailor your program accordingly. Similarly, if you encounter challenges or setbacks, communicate them promptly to receive appropriate support and adjustments to your plan.

2. **Regular Check-Ins:** Schedule regular check-ins with your coach to discuss progress, address any issues, and adjust your training plan as

needed. These check-ins provide an opportunity to review your achievements, set new goals, and make necessary modifications to your program. Consistent communication ensures that both you and your coach remain aligned and focused on achieving your fitness objectives.

3. **Provide Feedback:** Give constructive feedback to your coach about your training experience. If certain exercises or routines are not working for you, or if you have preferences for different types of workouts, share this feedback. This allows your coach to make adjustments that better suit your needs and preferences, enhancing your overall experience and effectiveness of the program.

4. **Set Clear Expectations:** Establish clear expectations for your coaching relationship. Discuss how often you expect to communicate, what level of support you need, and how you prefer to receive feedback. Setting these expectations ensures that both you and your coach are on the same page and can work together effectively.

5. **Use Technology for Communication:** Take advantage of technology to facilitate communication with your coach. Many coaches use apps, messaging platforms, or online portals to share workout plans, track progress, and provide feedback. Utilizing these tools can streamline

communication and make it easier to stay connected, especially if you have a busy schedule or prefer virtual interactions.

6. **Stay Engaged and Responsive:** Be proactive and engaged in your coaching relationship. Respond promptly to messages from your coach, participate actively in sessions, and follow through on recommendations. This engagement demonstrates your commitment to the process and helps your coach provide the best possible support.

7. **Discuss Challenges and Adjustments:** If you encounter any challenges or difficulties, discuss them with your coach. Whether it's a lack of motivation, an injury, or a change in your schedule, addressing these issues openly allows your coach to help you navigate them and make necessary adjustments to your plan.

By fostering effective communication and leveraging the support of your coach, you can enhance your motivation, maintain accountability, and achieve your fitness goals more efficiently. A well-structured coaching relationship provides the guidance, encouragement, and expertise needed to succeed on your fitness journey.

# The Impact of Coaching on Motivation and Accountability

## How a Coach Can Help You Stay Motivated

1. **Personalized Goal Setting:** A fitness coach plays a crucial role in setting realistic and personalized goals that align with your aspirations and current fitness level. By breaking down larger goals into smaller, achievable milestones, a coach helps you stay focused and motivated. For instance, if your primary goal is to lose 20 pounds, a coach might set monthly targets such as losing 2 pounds each month. This incremental approach keeps you motivated as you experience regular progress and celebrate small victories along the way.

2. **Customized Workouts:** A coach designs tailored workout programs that match your individual needs, preferences, and fitness levels. This personalization not only enhances the effectiveness of your training but also keeps you engaged. For example, if you enjoy high-intensity interval training (HIIT) but find weightlifting tedious, a coach might incorporate HIIT into your routine while gradually introducing weightlifting exercises in a way that feels manageable and interesting.

3. **Regular Progress Tracking:** Tracking progress is a powerful motivator, and a coach provides regular assessments to measure your achievements. By monitoring key metrics such as weight, strength, endurance, or flexibility, a coach helps you visualize your progress and stay motivated. This ongoing feedback allows you to see the tangible results of your efforts and reinforces your commitment to your fitness goals.

4. **Encouragement and Support:** A coach offers consistent encouragement and emotional support throughout your fitness journey. They celebrate your successes, provide constructive feedback, and help you overcome obstacles. For instance, if you hit a plateau or face a challenging period, your coach's support and reassurance can boost your morale and keep you motivated to push through difficult times.

5. **Structured Routine and Accountability:** Having scheduled sessions with a coach creates a structured routine and ensures accountability. Knowing that you have an appointment with your coach can motivate you to adhere to your workout plan and make healthier choices. This regular commitment helps maintain consistency, which is essential for long-term success. For example, if you have a session planned for three times a week, you're

more likely to stay committed to your training schedule compared to a self-guided plan without set appointments.

6. **Education and Inspiration:** A coach educates you about fitness principles, nutrition, and effective training techniques. This knowledge not only empowers you to make informed decisions but also inspires you to continue your fitness journey. For instance, learning about the benefits of strength training or understanding how proper nutrition supports recovery can motivate you to incorporate these practices into your routine.

## Strategies for Effective Communication with Your Coach

1. **Open and Honest Dialogue:** Effective communication begins with openness and honesty. Clearly express your goals, preferences, and any concerns you may have. If you have specific fitness goals, share them with your coach so they can tailor your program accordingly. Similarly, if you encounter challenges or setbacks, communicate them promptly to receive appropriate support and adjustments to your plan.

2. **Regular Check-Ins:** Schedule regular check-ins with your coach to discuss progress, address any issues, and adjust your training plan as

needed. These check-ins provide an opportunity to review your achievements, set new goals, and make necessary modifications to your program. Consistent communication ensures that both you and your coach remain aligned and focused on achieving your fitness objectives.

3.  **Provide Feedback:** Give constructive feedback to your coach about your training experience. If certain exercises or routines are not working for you, or if you have preferences for different types of workouts, share this feedback. This allows your coach to make adjustments that better suit your needs and preferences, enhancing your overall experience and effectiveness of the program.

4.  **Set Clear Expectations:** Establish clear expectations for your coaching relationship. Discuss how often you expect to communicate, what level of support you need, and how you prefer to receive feedback. Setting these expectations ensures that both you and your coach are on the same page and can work together effectively.

5.  **Use Technology for Communication:** Take advantage of technology to facilitate communication with your coach. Many coaches use apps, messaging platforms, or online portals to share workout plans, track progress, and provide feedback. Utilizing these tools can streamline

communication and make it easier to stay connected, especially if you have a busy schedule or prefer virtual interactions.

6. **Stay Engaged and Responsive:** Be proactive and engaged in your coaching relationship. Respond promptly to messages from your coach, participate actively in sessions, and follow through on recommendations. This engagement demonstrates your commitment to the process and helps your coach provide the best possible support.

7. **Discuss Challenges and Adjustments:** If you encounter any challenges or difficulties, discuss them with your coach. Whether it's a lack of motivation, an injury, or a change in your schedule, addressing these issues openly allows your coach to help you navigate them and make necessary adjustments to your plan.

By fostering effective communication and leveraging the support of your coach, you can enhance your motivation, maintain accountability, and achieve your fitness goals more efficiently. A well-structured coaching relationship provides the guidance, encouragement, and expertise needed to succeed on your fitness journey.

# The Evolution of Coaching Methods

How Coaching Has Changed with New Fitness Trends and Research

Coaching has undergone significant transformations over the years, driven by advances in fitness research, technology, and evolving trends in exercise and wellness. Here's how coaching methods have evolved:

1.  **Integration of Science and Data:** Modern coaching is increasingly informed by scientific research and data analytics. Coaches now use evidence-based practices to design personalized training programs that optimize performance and reduce the risk of injury. For instance, contemporary coaches rely on heart rate monitors, wearable fitness trackers, and biomechanical assessments to gather data on an individual's physical responses to exercise. This data helps in fine-tuning workouts and tracking progress with greater precision.

2.  **Emphasis on Functional Training:** Traditional coaching often focused on isolated strength exercises and traditional cardio workouts. Modern coaching, however, emphasizes functional training—exercises that mimic everyday movements and improve overall functionality. This approach aims to enhance strength, balance,

and coordination in a way that translates to better performance in daily activities. For example, modern trainers might incorporate exercises like kettlebell swings, medicine ball slams, and TRX suspension training into their programs to improve functional strength and mobility.

3. **Personalized and Holistic Approach:** Today's coaching methods prioritize a holistic view of fitness that includes not only exercise but also nutrition, mental health, and lifestyle factors. Coaches are increasingly focusing on creating comprehensive plans that address all aspects of an individual's well-being. This might involve personalized meal plans, stress management techniques, and sleep optimization strategies alongside tailored workout routines. This holistic approach recognizes that fitness is not just about physical exercise but also about overall health and wellness.

4. **Use of Technology:** The integration of technology into coaching has revolutionized the field. Coaches now utilize various digital tools to enhance their methods. Online coaching platforms, virtual training sessions, and fitness apps have made it possible for individuals to receive coaching remotely. These technologies allow for real-time feedback, remote tracking of progress, and virtual support, making coaching more accessible

and convenient. For example, virtual coaching platforms like Trainerize or MyFitnessPal offer interactive features for tracking workouts, nutrition, and communication with coaches.

5. **Focus on Mental Conditioning:** Modern coaching recognizes the importance of mental conditioning alongside physical training. Coaches now incorporate techniques such as mindfulness, visualization, and mental resilience training into their programs. This focus on mental aspects helps individuals develop a positive mindset, manage stress, and enhance overall performance. For instance, coaches might use guided imagery exercises to help athletes visualize successful performance or teach mindfulness techniques to improve focus and reduce anxiety.

6. **Evidence-Based Practices:** Contemporary coaches are increasingly relying on evidence-based practices to inform their methods. This means using strategies and interventions that have been validated through scientific research. For example, the use of high-intensity interval training (HIIT) has gained popularity due to its proven effectiveness in improving cardiovascular fitness and burning fat. Coaches are now more likely to incorporate such research-backed methods into

their programs to ensure that clients benefit from the latest advancements in fitness science.

## Examples of Traditional Versus Modern Coaching Techniques

**Traditional Coaching Techniques:**

1. **Generalized Workout Plans:** Traditional coaching often involved one-size-fits-all workout plans that were not tailored to individual needs. These plans might have included basic strength training routines and cardio exercises without considering personal goals or fitness levels.

2. **Limited Use of Technology:** Coaches in the past relied on basic tools and methods, such as paper workout logs and verbal instructions. There was limited use of technology for tracking progress or providing real-time feedback.

3. **Focus on Isolated Strength Training:** Traditional coaching emphasized isolated strength exercises, such as bicep curls and leg presses, with less emphasis on functional movements or compound exercises.

4. **Standardized Nutritional Advice:** Nutritional guidance in traditional coaching often involved generic recommendations, such as "eat more

protein" or "cut out carbs," without considering individual dietary needs or preferences.

**Modern Coaching Techniques:**

1.  **Personalized and Data-Driven Programs:** Modern coaches create highly personalized workout plans based on individual assessments, including data from fitness trackers and health evaluations. This approach ensures that programs are tailored to specific goals, fitness levels, and preferences.

2.  **Technology Integration:** Contemporary coaching utilizes advanced technology, such as wearable devices, mobile apps, and virtual coaching platforms. These tools provide real-time feedback, track progress, and facilitate remote coaching.

3.  **Functional and Compound Exercises:** Modern coaching emphasizes functional and compound exercises that engage multiple muscle groups and improve overall functionality. Exercises like kettlebell swings, burpees, and functional circuits are commonly used to enhance strength, balance, and coordination.

4.  **Holistic and Evidence-Based Approach:** Modern coaching adopts a holistic approach that includes not only exercise but also nutrition, mental conditioning, and lifestyle factors. Evidence-based

practices are incorporated to ensure that clients benefit from scientifically validated methods.

5. **Mental Conditioning and Resilience Training:** Coaches now integrate mental conditioning techniques, such as mindfulness and visualization, to support psychological well-being and enhance performance. This focus on mental aspects complements physical training and helps individuals achieve their goals.

By understanding the evolution of coaching methods, individuals can appreciate how advancements in fitness science, technology, and holistic approaches have shaped modern coaching practices. Embracing these contemporary techniques can lead to more effective, personalized, and comprehensive fitness solutions.

# Building a Support System for Fitness

How Family and Friends Can Support Your Fitness Journey

Building a solid support system is crucial for achieving and maintaining fitness goals. Family and friends play a significant role in this journey, offering motivation, encouragement, and practical help. Here's how they can support you:

1. **Encouragement and Motivation:** Family and friends can provide essential encouragement and motivation, especially during challenging times. Their support can come in the form of words of affirmation, celebrating milestones, or simply being present during workouts. For example, a friend who regularly checks in on your progress can help keep you accountable and motivated. When your family understands and supports your fitness goals, they can create a positive environment that fosters your commitment to exercise and healthy eating.

2. **Shared Activities:** Engaging in fitness activities together can strengthen relationships and make working out more enjoyable. Family outings that involve physical activity, like hiking, biking, or

playing sports, can be both fun and beneficial. Similarly, friends who join you for workout classes or running sessions can help you stay consistent. The camaraderie and shared experiences not only make fitness more enjoyable but also provide additional motivation to stick to your routine.

3.  **Practical Support:** Family and friends can offer practical support that makes it easier to integrate fitness into your life. This might include helping with childcare, preparing healthy meals, or offering to join you in meal planning and grocery shopping. For instance, a partner who helps with cooking nutritious meals can make it easier to adhere to a healthy diet. Additionally, having a workout buddy or a supportive spouse can help you stay committed to your fitness goals by sharing the responsibility of maintaining a healthy lifestyle.

4.  **Accountability:** Having a support system that keeps you accountable is a key factor in long-term success. Family members or friends who regularly check on your progress can help you stay on track. Accountability partners can also provide motivation and encouragement when you're tempted to skip a workout or deviate from your nutrition plan. For example, if you have a friend who's also working towards fitness goals,

you can check in with each other, share updates, and celebrate successes together.

5. **Understanding and Patience:** Achieving fitness goals often requires time and effort, and having supportive family and friends who understand this can be invaluable. Their patience and empathy can help you navigate setbacks and maintain a positive attitude. If you encounter obstacles or need to adjust your goals, having a supportive network that listens and provides constructive feedback can make a significant difference. For example, if you're facing a tough week at work and struggle to find time for exercise, understanding friends who offer encouragement and flexibility can help you get back on track.

## The Role of Support Groups and Communities in Achieving Fitness Goals

Support groups and communities offer additional layers of support that can significantly enhance your fitness journey. These groups provide a sense of belonging, shared experiences, and collective motivation. Here's how they contribute to achieving fitness goals:

1. **Sense of Belonging:** Joining a fitness support group or community can create a strong sense of belonging and connection. Being part of a group

with similar fitness goals fosters camaraderie and mutual support. Whether it's an online forum, a local running club, or a gym class, these communities provide a space where you can share experiences, seek advice, and find encouragement. For example, participating in a local fitness group or an online community can help you feel connected and less isolated in your fitness journey.

2. **Shared Knowledge and Resources:** Support groups often provide access to valuable knowledge, resources, and expertise. Members can share tips, strategies, and experiences that may be beneficial for your fitness journey. For instance, a running club might offer advice on improving running technique, finding suitable gear, or setting realistic goals. Similarly, online fitness communities might provide access to workout plans, nutrition advice, and motivational content that can help you stay informed and inspired.

3. **Group Accountability:** Being part of a fitness group or community can enhance accountability and commitment. Regular group meetings, challenges, or events create opportunities for you to stay engaged and track progress. For example, a group that organizes weekly workouts or monthly fitness challenges can help you maintain

consistency and stay motivated. The collective goals and shared experiences within the group contribute to a sense of responsibility and drive.

4.  **Motivation and Inspiration:** Support groups and communities can serve as a powerful source of motivation and inspiration. Hearing about others' successes, overcoming challenges, and achieving goals can be incredibly motivating. For instance, seeing fellow members reach their milestones or share their fitness journeys can inspire you to push through obstacles and stay dedicated to your goals. This positive reinforcement and shared enthusiasm contribute to a more dynamic and engaging fitness experience.

5.  **Emotional Support:** Fitness journeys can be accompanied by emotional highs and lows, and having access to a supportive community can provide crucial emotional support. Support groups offer a space where you can share your struggles, receive encouragement, and find understanding. For example, if you're facing a setback or struggling with motivation, a supportive community can offer empathy, practical advice, and encouragement to help you overcome challenges and keep moving forward.

In summary, building a support system for fitness involves leveraging the encouragement and practical help of family and friends, as well as engaging with support groups and communities. Both personal relationships and collective networks contribute to a more successful and fulfilling fitness journey by offering motivation, accountability, and a sense of belonging.

# Building a Support System for Fitness

## How Family and Friends Can Support Your Fitness Journey

Building a solid support system is crucial for achieving and maintaining fitness goals. Family and friends play a significant role in this journey, offering motivation, encouragement, and practical help. Here's how they can support you:

1. **Encouragement and Motivation:** Family and friends can provide essential encouragement and motivation, especially during challenging times. Their support can come in the form of words of affirmation, celebrating milestones, or simply being present during workouts. For example, a friend who regularly checks in on your progress can help keep you accountable and motivated. When your family understands and supports your fitness goals, they can create a positive environment that fosters your commitment to exercise and healthy eating.

2. **Shared Activities:** Engaging in fitness activities together can strengthen relationships and make working out more enjoyable. Family outings that involve physical activity, like hiking, biking, or

playing sports, can be both fun and beneficial. Similarly, friends who join you for workout classes or running sessions can help you stay consistent. The camaraderie and shared experiences not only make fitness more enjoyable but also provide additional motivation to stick to your routine.

3.  **Practical Support:** Family and friends can offer practical support that makes it easier to integrate fitness into your life. This might include helping with childcare, preparing healthy meals, or offering to join you in meal planning and grocery shopping. For instance, a partner who helps with cooking nutritious meals can make it easier to adhere to a healthy diet. Additionally, having a workout buddy or a supportive spouse can help you stay committed to your fitness goals by sharing the responsibility of maintaining a healthy lifestyle.

4.  **Accountability:** Having a support system that keeps you accountable is a key factor in long-term success. Family members or friends who regularly check on your progress can help you stay on track. Accountability partners can also provide motivation and encouragement when you're tempted to skip a workout or deviate from your nutrition plan. For example, if you have a friend who's also working towards fitness goals,

you can check in with each other, share updates, and celebrate successes together.

5. **Understanding and Patience:** Achieving fitness goals often requires time and effort, and having supportive family and friends who understand this can be invaluable. Their patience and empathy can help you navigate setbacks and maintain a positive attitude. If you encounter obstacles or need to adjust your goals, having a supportive network that listens and provides constructive feedback can make a significant difference. For example, if you're facing a tough week at work and struggle to find time for exercise, understanding friends who offer encouragement and flexibility can help you get back on track.

## The Role of Support Groups and Communities in Achieving Fitness Goals

Support groups and communities offer additional layers of support that can significantly enhance your fitness journey. These groups provide a sense of belonging, shared experiences, and collective motivation. Here's how they contribute to achieving fitness goals:

1. **Sense of Belonging:** Joining a fitness support group or community can create a strong sense of belonging and connection. Being part of a group

with similar fitness goals fosters camaraderie and mutual support. Whether it's an online forum, a local running club, or a gym class, these communities provide a space where you can share experiences, seek advice, and find encouragement. For example, participating in a local fitness group or an online community can help you feel connected and less isolated in your fitness journey.

2. **Shared Knowledge and Resources:** Support groups often provide access to valuable knowledge, resources, and expertise. Members can share tips, strategies, and experiences that may be beneficial for your fitness journey. For instance, a running club might offer advice on improving running technique, finding suitable gear, or setting realistic goals. Similarly, online fitness communities might provide access to workout plans, nutrition advice, and motivational content that can help you stay informed and inspired.

3. **Group Accountability:** Being part of a fitness group or community can enhance accountability and commitment. Regular group meetings, challenges, or events create opportunities for you to stay engaged and track progress. For example, a group that organizes weekly workouts or monthly fitness challenges can help you maintain

consistency and stay motivated. The collective goals and shared experiences within the group contribute to a sense of responsibility and drive.

4. **Motivation and Inspiration:** Support groups and communities can serve as a powerful source of motivation and inspiration. Hearing about others' successes, overcoming challenges, and achieving goals can be incredibly motivating. For instance, seeing fellow members reach their milestones or share their fitness journeys can inspire you to push through obstacles and stay dedicated to your goals. This positive reinforcement and shared enthusiasm contribute to a more dynamic and engaging fitness experience.

5. **Emotional Support:** Fitness journeys can be accompanied by emotional highs and lows, and having access to a supportive community can provide crucial emotional support. Support groups offer a space where you can share your struggles, receive encouragement, and find understanding. For example, if you're facing a setback or struggling with motivation, a supportive community can offer empathy, practical advice, and encouragement to help you overcome challenges and keep moving forward.

In summary, building a support system for fitness involves leveraging the encouragement and practical help of family and friends, as well as engaging with support groups and communities. Both personal relationships and collective networks contribute to a more successful and fulfilling fitness journey by offering motivation, accountability, and a sense of belonging.

# Leveraging Social Media and Online Communities

How Online Forums and Social Media Can Provide Support and Accountability

In today's digital age, social media and online communities have become powerful tools for enhancing fitness journeys. They offer unique opportunities for support, motivation, and accountability, making it easier to stay committed to your goals. Here's how online platforms can help:

1. **Access to Diverse Perspectives:** Online forums and social media platforms connect you with a vast array of individuals who share similar fitness goals or have achieved the success you're aspiring to. This diversity of perspectives allows you to learn from various experiences, gain insights into different fitness strategies, and adapt techniques that resonate with you. For instance, a Facebook group dedicated to weight loss might feature a range of success stories and advice that can inspire and guide your own journey.

2. **Real-Time Feedback and Interaction:** Social media platforms facilitate real-time interaction and feedback, allowing you to quickly share

updates, ask questions, and receive responses. This immediate engagement fosters a sense of community and support. For example, sharing your workout progress or challenges on Instagram can prompt encouragement and advice from followers and fellow fitness enthusiasts. The ability to interact in real-time helps maintain motivation and keeps you connected with others who are on similar journeys.

3. **Accountability Partners and Groups:** Online communities often feature accountability partners or groups that focus on specific fitness goals or challenges. Being part of an accountability group provides a structured way to stay committed and track progress. For instance, participating in a weekly challenge within a fitness group on Reddit or a monthly goal-setting thread on a fitness forum can help you stay on track and motivated. The shared commitment to goals within these groups fosters a supportive environment and encourages consistency.

4. **Access to Expert Advice and Resources:** Many online communities and social media platforms provide access to expert advice and resources that can enhance your fitness knowledge. Fitness influencers, trainers, and nutritionists often share valuable content, such as workout routines,

nutrition tips, and educational articles. Following these experts on platforms like YouTube or Twitter can provide you with reliable information and innovative ideas to incorporate into your fitness routine.

5. **Emotional Support and Encouragement:** Online communities offer emotional support and encouragement during times of struggle or frustration. When facing challenges or setbacks, connecting with others who understand your experiences can provide comfort and motivation. For example, joining a support group on a platform like Facebook or participating in discussions on a fitness forum can help you navigate difficult moments with empathy and encouragement from others who have faced similar challenges.

## Tips for Finding and Engaging with Supportive Online Fitness Communities

To make the most of online communities and social media for your fitness journey, consider the following tips for finding and engaging with supportive groups:

1. **Identify Your Goals and Interests:** Start by identifying your specific fitness goals and interests. Whether you're focused on weight loss, strength training, or a particular sport, look for communities that align with your objectives. For

instance, if your goal is to build muscle, search for bodybuilding groups or forums where members discuss muscle-building techniques and share workout routines.

2. **Research and Choose Reputable Platforms:** Research various platforms to find communities that are reputable and active. Some well-known options include Facebook groups, Reddit communities, and specialized fitness forums. Look for groups with a positive reputation, active discussions, and a supportive atmosphere. Reading reviews or recommendations can help you select the most suitable platforms for your needs.

3. **Participate Actively and Respectfully:** Engage actively in the communities you join by participating in discussions, sharing your experiences, and offering support to others. Respectful and constructive interactions contribute to a positive environment and help build meaningful connections. For example, contribute to discussions by sharing your progress, asking questions, and offering encouragement to fellow members.

4. **Set Boundaries and Manage Time:** While online communities can be a valuable source of support, it's important to set boundaries and manage

your time effectively. Avoid getting overwhelmed by excessive screen time or comparisons with others. Focus on engaging with communities that provide meaningful support and align with your personal fitness goals. Set specific times for online interactions to ensure a balanced approach to your fitness journey.

5.  **Be Selective About Influencers and Advice:** When following fitness influencers or experts on social media, be selective and critical of the advice you receive. Ensure that the information aligns with evidence-based practices and your personal goals. Look for credible sources and be wary of trends or advice that seem unrealistic or not backed by scientific research. For example, favor influencers who provide transparent and well-researched content over those promoting quick-fix solutions.

6.  **Build Genuine Connections:** Strive to build genuine connections with other members of the community. Authentic relationships can provide more meaningful support and encouragement. Engage with others by offering constructive feedback, celebrating their achievements, and seeking out accountability partners who share similar goals. For example, connect with someone who has similar fitness objectives and agree to check in with each other regularly to stay motivated.

In summary, leveraging social media and online communities can significantly enhance your fitness journey by providing access to diverse perspectives, real-time feedback, accountability partners, expert advice, and emotional support. By identifying your goals, choosing reputable platforms, participating actively, managing your time, and building genuine connections, you can maximize the benefits of online support and stay motivated on your path to fitness success.

# The Importance of Professional Support

## When to Seek Help from Nutritionists, Physiotherapists, and Other Professionals

In the pursuit of fitness and health, professional support plays a crucial role in guiding and optimizing your journey. While self-directed efforts are valuable, there are key situations where seeking help from experts such as nutritionists, physiotherapists, and other specialized professionals becomes essential. Here's when and why you might need their expertise:

1. **Facing Specific Health Issues or Conditions:** If you have specific health conditions or injuries, professional support is crucial. For example, if you're dealing with chronic knee pain or recovering from a sports injury, a physiotherapist can design a tailored rehabilitation program to address your unique needs and help you recover safely. Similarly, if you have diabetes or high blood pressure, consulting a nutritionist can ensure that your diet supports your medical requirements while contributing to overall well-being.

2. **Struggling with Plateaus or Lack of Progress:** When your fitness progress stalls or you hit a plateau

despite consistent efforts, seeking professional guidance can provide a fresh perspective. A fitness coach or personal trainer can analyze your current routine, identify potential gaps, and introduce new strategies to help you break through barriers. For instance, if you've been struggling to gain muscle mass, a personal trainer can adjust your workout regimen and nutritional intake to stimulate growth and progress.

3. **Need for Specialized Knowledge:** Certain fitness goals or health conditions require specialized knowledge that may go beyond general advice. For example, if you're preparing for a bodybuilding competition or an endurance event like a marathon, working with a specialized coach who has experience in these areas can provide insights and strategies specific to your goals. A sports nutritionist, for instance, can help optimize your diet to enhance performance and recovery for competitive sports.

4. **Improving Technique and Preventing Injuries:** Proper technique and form are essential to prevent injuries and maximize workout effectiveness. A physiotherapist or experienced personal trainer can assess your exercise technique and make corrections to ensure you're performing movements safely and effectively. This is especially

important when performing complex exercises like Olympic lifts or high-intensity interval training (HIIT), where improper form can lead to injuries.

5. **Customized Nutrition Planning:** Nutrition plays a critical role in achieving fitness goals, and a nutritionist can offer personalized dietary plans based on your individual needs, goals, and preferences. Whether you're aiming to lose weight, build muscle, or improve overall health, a nutritionist can create a meal plan that aligns with your objectives, helps you meet your nutritional needs, and supports your fitness regimen.

6. **Addressing Emotional or Psychological Barriers:** Fitness journeys often involve psychological challenges such as motivation, stress, or body image issues. A sports psychologist or counselor can provide support to address these emotional barriers and develop strategies to enhance mental resilience and focus. For example, if you're experiencing anxiety related to performance or body image, a sports psychologist can help you develop coping strategies and a positive mindset.

## How Professional Support Can Enhance Your Fitness Journey

Incorporating professional support into your fitness journey can offer numerous benefits, enhancing both the effectiveness and enjoyment of your efforts. Here's how professional guidance can make a significant impact:

1. **Expert Guidance and Personalization:** Professionals bring a wealth of knowledge and experience that can tailor your fitness and nutrition plans to your specific needs. For example, a nutritionist can assess your dietary habits, lifestyle, and health goals to create a customized meal plan that not only meets your nutritional requirements but also aligns with your preferences and lifestyle. This personalized approach ensures that you're following a plan that's designed specifically for you, increasing the likelihood of achieving your goals.

2. **Structured and Evidence-Based Approaches:** Professionals use evidence-based practices to design and implement effective strategies. For instance, a physiotherapist will use proven rehabilitation techniques and assessments to address injuries and improve mobility. Similarly, a certified personal trainer will utilize scientifically backed exercise programs to optimize performance and results. This structured approach helps you avoid guesswork and ensures that your efforts are aligned with best practices in the field.

3. **Accountability and Motivation:** Working with professionals provides a layer of accountability that can enhance your motivation. Scheduled sessions with a personal trainer or regular check-ins with a nutritionist create a commitment that encourages adherence to your plan. For example, knowing that you have a training session or consultation scheduled can motivate you to stay consistent with your workouts and dietary choices. Additionally, professionals offer encouragement and support to help you stay motivated during challenging times.

4. **Efficient and Safe Progression:** Professionals help you progress efficiently and safely by providing guidance on appropriate intensity, volume, and recovery. A fitness coach can design a progressive workout program that gradually increases in complexity and intensity, ensuring you're continually challenged without risking overtraining or injury. This structured progression helps you achieve your goals more effectively while minimizing the risk of setbacks.

5. **Holistic Approach to Wellness:** Many professionals, such as integrative health coaches or sports dietitians, take a holistic approach to wellness that encompasses various aspects of your health. This approach considers factors such as sleep, stress management, and overall lifestyle in

addition to exercise and nutrition. For example, a holistic health coach might work with you on developing strategies to improve sleep quality, manage stress, and incorporate healthy habits into your daily routine, leading to overall better health and well-being.

6. **Learning and Skill Development:** Working with experts provides opportunities for learning and skill development. You can gain valuable insights into effective exercise techniques, nutritional strategies, and injury prevention methods. For instance, a personal trainer can teach you proper lifting techniques and how to perform exercises with correct form, which not only enhances your workout effectiveness but also equips you with knowledge for future fitness endeavors.

In summary, professional support plays a vital role in enhancing your fitness journey by offering personalized guidance, evidence-based approaches, accountability, safe progression, and a holistic view of wellness. By seeking help from nutritionists, physiotherapists, and other experts, you can optimize your efforts, address specific challenges, and achieve your fitness goals more effectively and sustainably.

## How Recovery Impacts Muscle Growth and Overall Fitness

Recovery is a critical yet often overlooked component of a successful fitness regimen. It plays a crucial role in muscle growth, overall fitness, and long-term health. Here's a detailed look at how recovery affects these aspects:

1. **Muscle Growth:** During intense exercise, particularly strength training, muscle fibers experience microscopic damage. This is a normal part of the process known as muscle hypertrophy, where muscle fibers repair and grow stronger in response to the stress. Recovery allows the body to repair this damage, leading to muscle growth. Without adequate recovery, this repair process is compromised, which can hinder muscle growth and lead to decreased strength and performance.

2. **Prevention of Overtraining:** Overtraining syndrome occurs when the body is subjected to excessive exercise without sufficient recovery, leading to decreased performance, fatigue, and increased risk of injury. Adequate recovery helps prevent overtraining by allowing the body to repair

and adapt to the stresses of exercise. This balance between training and recovery is essential for maintaining optimal performance and avoiding burnout.

3. **Restoration of Energy Stores:** Exercise depletes the body's energy stores, particularly glycogen, which is the primary fuel source for high-intensity activities. Recovery periods are essential for replenishing these glycogen stores. Proper recovery strategies, including carbohydrate intake, help restore energy levels and ensure that the body is ready for subsequent workouts.

4. **Hormonal Balance:** Intense exercise can impact hormonal levels, including stress hormones like cortisol. Chronic high levels of cortisol due to insufficient recovery can negatively affect muscle growth, immune function, and overall health. Recovery helps regulate hormonal balance, allowing the body to return to a state of equilibrium and maintain optimal physiological function.

5. **Reduction of Muscle Soreness:** Delayed onset muscle soreness (DOMS) is a common experience after intense exercise, especially when trying new workouts or increasing intensity. Recovery techniques such as stretching, massage, and proper hydration can help alleviate muscle soreness and

stiffness, making it easier to continue with regular exercise.

## Techniques for Effective Recovery

Effective recovery involves multiple strategies that address various aspects of physical and mental rejuvenation. Here are some key techniques:

1. **Rest and Sleep:** Rest is the cornerstone of recovery. Ensuring you get sufficient quality sleep each night is vital for muscle repair, energy restoration, and overall health. During deep sleep stages, the body releases growth hormones that facilitate muscle growth and repair. Aim for 7-9 hours of sleep per night and consider implementing sleep hygiene practices such as maintaining a consistent sleep schedule, creating a restful environment, and avoiding screens before bedtime.

2. **Nutrition:** Proper nutrition is essential for effective recovery. After exercise, the body needs nutrients to repair muscle tissues and replenish energy stores. A post-workout meal or snack that combines protein and carbohydrates can accelerate recovery. For example, a smoothie made with protein powder, fruit, and yogurt provides the necessary nutrients for muscle repair and glycogen replenishment. Additionally, staying hydrated is crucial as water supports digestion, nutrient transport, and overall metabolic processes.

3. **Active Recovery:** Active recovery involves engaging in low-intensity activities that promote blood flow and aid in muscle recovery. Examples include walking, light cycling, or gentle stretching. Active recovery helps flush out metabolic waste products from intense exercise and delivers nutrients to muscle tissues more efficiently. Incorporating activities like yoga or foam rolling into your routine can also enhance flexibility and reduce muscle tightness.

4. **Massage and Foam Rolling:** Massage therapy and foam rolling can alleviate muscle soreness and improve circulation. Massage helps relax muscles, reduce tension, and promote relaxation, while foam rolling (self-myofascial release) targets specific muscle groups to release tightness and improve range of motion. Both techniques can be particularly beneficial after intense training sessions or competitions.

5. **Hydration:** Proper hydration is crucial for recovery as it aids in nutrient transport, waste removal, and maintaining electrolyte balance. Drinking enough water throughout the day helps prevent dehydration and supports overall bodily functions. After intense exercise, consider consuming electrolyte-rich beverages or adding a pinch of salt to your water to replenish lost electrolytes.

6. **Gradual Return to Intensity:** When resuming exercise after a period of rest or recovery, gradually increasing intensity is important to avoid injury and overtraining. Start with lower intensity and gradually progress to more challenging workouts as your body adapts. This approach allows for a smoother transition back to regular training and reduces the risk of setbacks.

7. **Mindfulness and Stress Management:** Mental recovery is as important as physical recovery. High levels of stress can impact your overall well-being and hinder recovery. Techniques such as mindfulness, meditation, and relaxation exercises can help manage stress, improve mental clarity, and support a balanced approach to fitness and recovery.

In summary, recovery is a vital component of any fitness regimen, playing a key role in muscle growth, preventing overtraining, restoring energy stores, balancing hormones, and reducing muscle soreness. By incorporating effective recovery techniques such as adequate rest, proper nutrition, active recovery, massage, hydration, gradual intensity, and stress management, you can enhance your overall fitness and well-being, leading to improved performance and long-term health.

# Balancing Cardio and Strength Training

**Creating a Balanced Workout Plan**

Balancing cardio and strength training is essential for achieving a well-rounded fitness regimen that enhances overall health, improves physical performance, and supports various fitness goals. Here's a comprehensive guide on how to create a balanced workout plan that incorporates both types of exercise, along with the benefits of this approach.

## Understanding Cardio and Strength Training

**Cardiovascular Training (Cardio):** Cardio exercises are activities that increase your heart rate and improve cardiovascular endurance. Common forms of cardio include running, cycling, swimming, and brisk walking. The primary benefits of cardio include enhanced heart health, improved lung capacity, and increased calorie burn, which can aid in weight management and overall fitness.

**Strength Training (Resistance Training):** Strength training focuses on building muscle strength, size, and endurance by working against resistance. This can be achieved through exercises like weightlifting, bodyweight exercises (e.g., push-ups, squats), and resistance band exercises. Strength training benefits include increased muscle mass, enhanced metabolic rate, improved bone density, and better functional strength for daily activities.

## Creating a Balanced Workout Plan

1. **Assess Your Fitness Goals:** Your fitness goals will determine the emphasis you place on cardio versus strength training. For example:

   ➤ **Weight Loss:** If your primary goal is weight loss, a higher emphasis on cardio may be beneficial for burning calories, complemented by strength training to build muscle and boost metabolism.

   ➤ **Muscle Building:** If you aim to build muscle, prioritize strength training with some cardio to maintain cardiovascular health and manage body fat.

   ➤ **General Fitness:** For overall health and fitness, a balanced approach with equal attention to both cardio and strength training can provide comprehensive benefits.

2. **Design Your Weekly Workout Schedule:** Incorporate both cardio and strength training into your weekly routine to achieve a balanced workout plan. A sample weekly schedule might look like this:

   • **Monday:** Full-body strength training

- **Tuesday:** Cardio (e.g., running or cycling)

- **Wednesday:** Rest or active recovery (e.g., yoga or light stretching)

- **Thursday:** Strength training (focus on different muscle groups)

- **Friday:** Cardio (e.g., interval training or swimming)

- **Saturday:** Strength training or functional training

- **Sunday:** Rest or low-intensity activity (e.g., walking or leisure biking)

3. **Balance Cardio and Strength Sessions:** Ensure that your workouts are balanced by incorporating both cardio and strength training within the same week. Aim to include at least two to three strength training sessions and two to three cardio sessions each week. Adjust the intensity and duration based on your fitness level and goals.

4. **Combine Cardio and Strength in One Session:** If time constraints or preferences make it challenging to separate cardio and strength training, consider combining them in one workout session. For instance:

- **Circuit Training:** Alternate between strength exercises (e.g., squats, push-ups) and cardio intervals (e.g., jumping jacks, high knees) within the same workout.

- **HIIT (High-Intensity Interval Training):** Incorporate short bursts of high-intensity cardio exercises with strength exercises for a time-efficient and effective workout.

5. **Allow for Recovery:** Recovery is crucial to avoid overtraining and injury. Incorporate rest days and ensure that you're allowing sufficient time for muscle recovery between strength training sessions. Active recovery days, where you engage in low-intensity activities like walking or stretching, can also be beneficial.

6. **Monitor Progress and Adjust:** Regularly assess your progress and adjust your workout plan as needed. If you find that you're not achieving your goals or if you're experiencing fatigue, modify the balance between cardio and strength training or adjust the intensity and duration of your workouts.

## The Benefits of Combining Cardio and Strength Training

1. **Improved Overall Fitness:** Combining cardio and strength training provides a comprehensive approach to fitness that improves cardiovascular

health, builds muscle strength, and enhances overall endurance. This balanced approach supports better physical performance and functional fitness.

2. **Increased Metabolic Rate:** Strength training builds muscle mass, which increases your resting metabolic rate (RMR). This means you burn more calories at rest, which can support weight management. Cardio complements this by increasing calorie expenditure during exercise.

3. **Enhanced Weight Management:** A combination of cardio and strength training is effective for managing body weight. Cardio helps burn calories and reduce body fat, while strength training builds muscle and boosts metabolism. Together, they create a balanced approach to achieving and maintaining a healthy weight.

4. **Better Functional Strength and Endurance:** Cardio improves endurance and stamina, allowing you to engage in physical activities for longer periods without fatigue. Strength training enhances muscle strength and power, contributing to better performance in daily tasks and physical activities.

5. **Reduced Risk of Injury:** Strength training improves muscle strength and joint stability, which

can reduce the risk of injuries. Combining this with cardio helps maintain cardiovascular health and supports overall fitness, making it easier to perform various physical activities safely.

6. **Enhanced Mental Health:** Both cardio and strength training have been shown to improve mental health by reducing stress, anxiety, and symptoms of depression. A balanced approach can provide holistic benefits for both physical and mental well-being.

In summary, creating a balanced workout plan that includes both cardio and strength training is essential for achieving comprehensive fitness benefits. By assessing your goals, designing a well-structured schedule, incorporating both types of exercise, allowing for recovery, and adjusting based on progress, you can optimize your fitness regimen and enjoy the diverse benefits of a well-rounded approach to exercise.

# Mental Health and Fitness

## The Relationship Between Mental Health and Physical Fitness

The link between mental health and physical fitness is well-established, with numerous studies showing that regular physical activity plays a crucial role in enhancing mental well-being. This connection is not merely anecdotal; it's supported by scientific research that reveals how exercise impacts the brain and emotions. Here's an in-depth look at how physical fitness influences mental health and practical strategies for leveraging exercise to improve mental well-being.

## How Exercise Impacts Mental Health

1. **Release of Endorphins:** Exercise stimulates the release of endorphins, often referred to as "feel-good" hormones. These chemicals act as natural painkillers and mood elevators. Regular physical activity can lead to a long-lasting improvement in mood, reducing feelings of depression and anxiety.

2. **Reduction in Stress:** Physical activity helps to lower levels of cortisol, the body's primary stress

hormone. By reducing cortisol levels, exercise can help mitigate the effects of stress and promote a sense of calm. Activities like walking, jogging, or yoga are particularly effective in reducing stress levels.

3. **Improved Sleep:** Exercise has been shown to improve the quality of sleep by helping to regulate sleep patterns. Better sleep contributes to improved mood and cognitive function. Regular physical activity can help alleviate insomnia and other sleep disorders, leading to better mental health.

4. **Enhanced Cognitive Function:** Regular physical activity boosts brain function by increasing blood flow to the brain. This can improve cognitive functions such as memory, attention, and problem-solving skills. Activities that require coordination and strategic thinking, like team sports, can further enhance cognitive abilities.

5. **Increased Self-Esteem:** Engaging in regular exercise can improve self-esteem and body image. Achieving fitness goals, whether it's running a certain distance or lifting heavier weights, can lead to a sense of accomplishment and increased self-worth.

6. **Social Interaction:** Group exercises and team sports offer opportunities for social interaction,

which can be beneficial for mental health. Building relationships and feeling part of a community can reduce feelings of isolation and improve overall emotional well-being.

## Strategies for Improving Mental Health Through Exercise

1. **Set Realistic Goals:** Setting achievable fitness goals can provide a sense of purpose and motivation. Start with small, manageable goals and gradually increase the difficulty as you progress. For example, begin with a 10-minute daily walk and gradually extend the duration or intensity.

2. **Choose Activities You Enjoy:** Engage in physical activities that you find enjoyable. Whether it's dancing, hiking, swimming, or playing a sport, finding something you love can make exercise feel less like a chore and more like a rewarding experience.

3. **Incorporate Mind-Body Practices:** Mind-body exercises such as yoga and Pilates not only improve physical fitness but also promote mental relaxation and mindfulness. These practices combine physical movement with breathing exercises and meditation, which can help reduce stress and enhance mental clarity.

4.  **Establish a Routine:** Consistency is key to reaping the mental health benefits of exercise. Establish a regular workout routine that fits your schedule and stick to it. Consistent exercise helps to stabilize mood and reduce symptoms of anxiety and depression over time.

5.  **Engage in Social Exercise:** Participate in group fitness classes or team sports to combine the benefits of exercise with social interaction. Social exercise can enhance motivation, provide support, and offer a sense of belonging, all of which contribute to better mental health.

6.  **Practice Mindfulness During Exercise:** Incorporate mindfulness techniques into your workouts. Focus on your breathing, the sensations in your body, and the present moment. Mindful exercise can help you stay grounded and reduce mental clutter, enhancing the overall mental health benefits.

7.  **Use Exercise as a Stress Management Tool:** Whenever you feel overwhelmed or stressed, use exercise as a tool to manage your emotions. A brisk walk, a short run, or a workout session can help you clear your mind and gain perspective on stressful situations.

8. **Track Your Progress:** Keep a journal or use an app to track your exercise routine and monitor your progress. Recording your achievements can provide a sense of accomplishment and motivation, contributing to improved mental well-being.

9. **Seek Professional Guidance:** If you're struggling with mental health issues, consider seeking guidance from a mental health professional or a fitness coach. They can help you develop a personalized exercise plan that addresses both your physical and mental health needs.

10. **Be Patient with Yourself:** Recognize that improving mental health through exercise is a gradual process. Be patient with yourself and celebrate small victories along the way. Understanding that progress takes time can help you stay motivated and committed to your fitness journey.

In summary, the relationship between mental health and physical fitness is profound, with exercise offering numerous benefits for mental well-being. By incorporating regular physical activity into your routine and adopting strategies that enhance both physical and mental health, you can improve your overall quality of life and achieve greater emotional balance.

## The Role of Fitness Apps and Wearables

### How Fitness Apps and Wearables Can Help Track Progress and Improve Performance

In the digital age, fitness apps and wearables have revolutionized the way we approach health and fitness. These technologies offer an array of tools to track progress, enhance performance, and achieve personal fitness goals. Here's an in-depth look at how these technologies work and their benefits:

1.  **Real-Time Tracking:** Fitness apps and wearables provide real-time tracking of various metrics such as heart rate, calories burned, distance traveled, and steps taken. This immediate feedback helps users stay aware of their performance and adjust their workouts accordingly. For example, a wearable like a Fitbit or an Apple Watch can monitor your heart rate throughout a run, allowing you to stay within your target heart rate zone for optimal cardiovascular benefits.

2.  **Data Analysis and Insights:** Fitness apps collect and analyze data over time, offering insights into trends and patterns in your activity. These insights can help you understand your progress, identify areas for improvement, and make informed decisions about your fitness routine. For instance, if a user notices a decline in their running pace over

several weeks, the app may suggest adjustments to their training plan or rest periods.

3. **Goal Setting and Motivation:** Fitness apps often include features for setting personal goals, such as daily step targets or weekly workout milestones. Many apps provide motivational features like reminders, achievement badges, and progress charts to keep users engaged and motivated. For example, an app might send a reminder to complete your daily workout or celebrate reaching a milestone with a virtual badge, helping to maintain motivation.

4. **Personalized Workouts:** Some fitness apps offer personalized workout plans based on your fitness level, goals, and preferences. By inputting data such as your fitness goals, current activity level, and available equipment, these apps can generate tailored workout routines that adjust as you progress. This customization ensures that workouts remain challenging and effective, aligning with your individual needs.

5. **Integration with Other Health Metrics:** Many fitness wearables and apps integrate with other health metrics, such as sleep patterns, stress levels, and nutrition. By providing a comprehensive view of your overall health, these tools help you understand how various factors influence your

fitness. For example, an app that tracks both sleep quality and exercise can offer insights into how your sleep affects your performance and recovery.

6. **Social Features and Community Engagement:** Fitness apps often include social features that allow users to connect with friends, join challenges, and participate in community forums. These social elements can enhance motivation and accountability by fostering a sense of community and friendly competition. For instance, participating in a step challenge with friends can encourage you to stay active and reach your daily step goals.

7. **Recovery and Injury Prevention:** Some apps and wearables offer features that help with recovery and injury prevention, such as tracking your recovery time between workouts and providing recommendations for stretching and mobility exercises. For example, an app might suggest specific stretches or foam rolling techniques to aid in muscle recovery after a strenuous workout.

8. **Health and Fitness Monitoring:** Advanced wearables can monitor a wide range of health indicators, including blood oxygen levels, ECG readings, and stress levels. This comprehensive monitoring allows users to gain deeper insights into their health and take proactive steps to address

any issues. For example, a wearable that tracks blood oxygen levels can alert users to potential respiratory concerns or irregularities.

## The Future of Fitness Technology and Its Potential Impact

The future of fitness technology promises even greater advancements, with innovations likely to transform how we approach health and fitness. Here are some emerging trends and their potential impact:

1. **AI and Machine Learning:** Artificial Intelligence (AI) and machine learning are expected to play a significant role in the future of fitness technology. AI-driven fitness apps and wearables could offer even more personalized recommendations by analyzing vast amounts of data and learning from user behavior. For example, AI might create highly individualized workout plans and dietary suggestions based on real-time feedback and historical data.

2. **Enhanced Wearable Technology:** Future wearables are likely to be more advanced, with improved sensors and capabilities for monitoring a wider range of health metrics. Innovations such as smart clothing with embedded sensors could provide detailed information about muscle activity, body temperature, and posture. This

enhanced technology could lead to more accurate assessments of physical performance and recovery.

3. **Virtual and Augmented Reality:** Virtual Reality (VR) and Augmented Reality (AR) are set to revolutionize the fitness experience by offering immersive workout environments and interactive training sessions. VR could create virtual fitness classes or simulations that make workouts more engaging, while AR might provide real-time feedback and guidance during exercises. For instance, an AR headset could project form corrections and exercise tips during a workout.

4. **Advanced Data Integration:** Future fitness technologies will likely offer more advanced integration with other health and wellness data sources, such as genetic information and environmental factors. This integration could provide a holistic view of an individual's health and fitness, leading to more precise and effective recommendations. For example, combining genetic data with fitness tracking could offer insights into optimal workout types and dietary needs.

5. **Personalized Nutrition and Supplements:** Advancements in technology may lead to more personalized nutrition and supplement recommendations based on individual data and

preferences. Wearables could track nutritional intake and provide tailored advice on how to optimize diet and supplementation for specific fitness goals. For example, an app might analyze your dietary habits and suggest personalized meal plans or supplements to enhance performance and recovery.

6. **Improved User Experience:** Future fitness technology is expected to offer a more seamless and intuitive user experience, with enhanced interfaces and streamlined interactions. This could include voice-activated controls, gesture recognition, and more interactive and user-friendly app designs. For instance, voice-activated fitness apps could allow users to start workouts, track progress, and receive feedback hands-free.

7. **Integration with Smart Home Technology:** Fitness technology will likely integrate with smart home devices, creating a connected and automated fitness environment. This integration could include features such as smart gym equipment that adjusts resistance based on your performance or a home assistant that provides workout reminders and guidance. For example, a smart treadmill might adjust speed and incline based on your fitness level and goals.

In summary, fitness apps and wearables are transforming the way we approach health and fitness by providing valuable tools for tracking progress, enhancing performance, and staying motivated. As technology continues to advance, the future of fitness promises even more innovative solutions that will further improve our ability to achieve and maintain optimal health and fitness.

# Nutrition Myths and Facts

## Common Myths About Nutrition and the Truths Behind Them

Nutrition is a field fraught with myths and misconceptions, often fueled by misinformation and a lack of scientific understanding. Here, we'll debunk some common nutrition myths and provide evidence-based truths to guide you toward making informed dietary choices.

### 1. Myth: Carbs Are Bad for You

**Fact:** Carbohydrates are not inherently bad; they are a primary source of energy for the body. The type and quality of carbohydrates you consume matter more than the quantity. Whole grains, fruits, and vegetables provide essential nutrients and fiber, which are beneficial for overall health. In contrast, refined carbohydrates, such as sugary snacks and white bread, can lead to weight gain and other health issues if consumed in excess.

**Example:** A diet rich in complex carbohydrates like quinoa, sweet potatoes, and beans supports sustained energy levels and provides essential vitamins and minerals. These carbs help fuel workouts, support brain function, and regulate blood sugar levels. On the other hand, a diet high in sugary cereals and pastries can lead to energy crashes and contribute to long-term health problems.

## 2.  Myth: All Fats Are Bad

**Fact:** Not all fats are created equal. While trans fats and excessive saturated fats can increase the risk of heart disease, unsaturated fats—found in sources like avocados, nuts, and olive oil—are beneficial. These healthy fats support brain function, hormone production, and cellular health. Omega-3 fatty acids, a type of polyunsaturated fat found in fatty fish, have anti-inflammatory properties and promote heart health.

**Example:** Incorporating avocados into your diet can provide healthy monounsaturated fats, which are linked to improved cholesterol levels and heart health. Similarly, eating a serving of salmon a few times a week ensures an adequate intake of omega-3 fatty acids, which can reduce inflammation and support cognitive function.

## 3.  Myth: Eating Late at Night Causes Weight Gain

**Fact:** Weight gain is primarily a result of consuming more calories than you expend, not the timing of your meals. What matters more is the overall quality and quantity of your diet throughout the day. Eating a balanced meal or snack before bed can help regulate blood sugar levels and prevent nighttime hunger.

**Example:** A light evening snack, such as Greek yogurt with berries, can help maintain stable blood sugar levels and prevent overeating at night. If you go to bed hungry, you may be more likely to experience disrupted sleep or wake up feeling ravenous, leading to less healthy food choices the next day.

### 4. Myth: Detox Diets Are Necessary for Cleansing Your Body

**Fact:** The human body is equipped with its own detoxification systems, primarily the liver and kidneys, which effectively filter and eliminate toxins. There is no scientific evidence to support the need for detox diets or cleanses to remove toxins. Instead, focus on a balanced diet rich in fruits, vegetables, and water to support your body's natural detoxification processes.

**Example:** Drinking plenty of water and eating a variety of colorful fruits and vegetables, such as leafy greens and berries, helps support liver and kidney function naturally. These foods provide essential nutrients and antioxidants that promote overall health without the need for restrictive detox diets.

### 5. Myth: Supplements Can Replace a Balanced Diet

**Fact:** While supplements can help fill nutritional gaps, they cannot replace the benefits of a balanced diet. Whole foods provide a range of nutrients, including fiber and phytochemicals, that supplements cannot fully replicate. A diet rich in diverse, nutrient-dense foods is essential for optimal health.

**Example:** Taking a vitamin C supplement is beneficial if you have a deficiency, but it should not replace consuming vitamin C-rich foods like oranges, strawberries, and bell peppers. These whole foods offer additional nutrients and health benefits beyond what a supplement can provide.

## 6.  Myth: All Calories Are Equal

**Fact:** Not all calories are created equal. The source of the calories you consume affects your overall health and how your body processes them. Nutrient-dense foods provide essential vitamins, minerals, and other beneficial compounds, while empty-calorie foods—high in sugar and low in nutrients—can lead to weight gain and poor health outcomes.

**Example:** A 200-calorie serving of almonds offers healthy fats, protein, fiber, and vitamins, while a 200-calorie serving of candy provides only sugar and empty calories. The almonds contribute to satiety, support muscle function, and provide essential nutrients, whereas the candy can lead to blood sugar spikes and lack of nutritional value.

## 7.  Myth: Protein Is Only for Bodybuilders

**Fact:** Protein is an essential macronutrient needed for various bodily functions, including muscle repair, immune system support, and hormone production. It is important for everyone, not just athletes or bodybuilders. Adequate protein intake supports overall health, helps maintain muscle mass, and aids in weight management.

**Example:** Including lean protein sources such as chicken, beans, and tofu in your diet helps repair tissues, support immune function, and promote satiety. Even if you're not lifting weights, protein plays a vital role in maintaining your body's structure and function.

## How to Discern Fact from Fiction in Dietary Advice

In the age of information overload, it can be challenging to separate fact from fiction in dietary advice. Here are some tips to help you discern reliable information:

1. **Check the Source:** Rely on information from reputable sources such as registered dietitians, nutritionists, and peer-reviewed scientific journals. Be cautious of advice from unverified websites, social media influencers, or those promoting commercial products.

2. **Look for Evidence:** Evidence-based information is supported by scientific research and clinical studies. Avoid claims that lack empirical support or are based on anecdotal evidence.

3. **Consider the Consensus:** Scientific consensus is reached when multiple studies and experts agree on a particular topic. Look for advice that aligns with established guidelines and recommendations from reputable health organizations.

4. **Be Skeptical of Quick Fixes:** Be wary of diets or supplements that promise rapid results or make extraordinary claims. Sustainable health improvements are typically achieved through gradual, evidence-based changes.

5. **Consult Professionals:** For personalized advice, consult with healthcare professionals or registered dietitians who can provide guidance based on your individual needs and health conditions.

By understanding and addressing these common myths and following these strategies for discerning reliable information, you can make informed dietary choices that support your health and well-being.

# Long-Term Fitness Strategies

Maintaining fitness and health over the long term requires more than just sticking to a temporary exercise program or diet. It involves cultivating habits that promote lifelong wellness, adapting to changes, and making fitness a sustainable part of your lifestyle. Here's how to build and sustain a long-term fitness strategy.

## How to Maintain Fitness and Health Over the Long Term

### 1. Set Realistic Goals and Expectations

Long-term fitness success starts with setting realistic, achievable goals. Rather than aiming for drastic changes, focus on incremental improvements that you can sustain. For instance, setting a goal to exercise three times a week for 30 minutes is more manageable and sustainable than committing to a daily two-hour workout.

### 2. Create a Balanced Routine

A balanced fitness routine includes a mix of cardiovascular exercise, strength training, and flexibility work. This variety ensures that you address different aspects of fitness, reduce the risk of overuse injuries, and keep workouts interesting. For example, you might alternate between running, weightlifting, and yoga throughout the week.

### 3. Build Healthy Habits

Incorporate fitness into your daily routine by creating healthy habits. This could involve scheduling workouts at the same time each day, preparing nutritious meals in advance, or finding an accountability partner. Consistency is key to making fitness a regular part of your life.

### 4. Monitor Progress and Adapt

Regularly track your progress to stay motivated and identify areas for improvement. This could involve keeping a workout journal, using a fitness app, or periodically reassessing your fitness levels. Be prepared to adapt your routine based on your progress, interests, and any new fitness goals you set.

### 5. Prioritize Recovery

Recovery is essential for long-term fitness. Ensure you get adequate rest between workouts, practice good sleep hygiene, and incorporate recovery techniques such as stretching, foam rolling, and proper nutrition. Allowing your body to recover helps prevent burnout and reduces the risk of injuries.

## 6. Stay Educated and Informed

Keep up with the latest fitness trends and research to stay informed about effective strategies and new developments. This knowledge can help you make better decisions about your fitness routine and adapt to changes in your body or lifestyle.

## 7. Maintain a Positive Attitude

A positive mindset can significantly impact your long-term success. Embrace setbacks as learning opportunities rather than failures. Celebrate small victories and stay focused on the benefits of maintaining a healthy lifestyle.

# Adapting Your Fitness Routine as Life Changes

Life is full of changes—whether it's starting a new job, having a baby, or dealing with aging—and your fitness routine may need to adapt accordingly. Here's how to make adjustments:

## 1. Adjust Workouts to Fit Your Schedule

Life changes often affect your availability for workouts. If you find yourself with less time, consider shorter, more efficient workouts like high-intensity interval training (HIIT). Alternatively, incorporate physical activity into your daily routine, such as walking or biking to work, or doing bodyweight exercises at home.

### 2.  Adapt to Physical Changes

As you age or experience physical changes, modify your routine to accommodate these changes. For example, older adults may need to focus more on strength training and flexibility to maintain muscle mass and joint health. If you experience an injury or health issue, work with a healthcare professional to adjust your routine accordingly.

### 3.  Incorporate Family-Friendly Activities

If family responsibilities impact your workout schedule, find ways to include physical activity in family time. Activities like hiking, biking, or playing sports with your family can be enjoyable and beneficial.

### 4.  Adjust Goals Based on New Priorities

As life circumstances evolve, your fitness goals may need to change. Reevaluate your goals periodically and adjust them based on your current priorities, such as preparing for a specific event, improving overall health, or managing stress.

### 5.  Seek Professional Guidance

When dealing with significant life changes or physical challenges, consider seeking guidance from a fitness professional or coach. They can help you create a customized plan that aligns with your new needs and goals.

## 6. Embrace Flexibility and Variety

To maintain long-term fitness, embrace flexibility and variety in your routine. Be open to trying new activities and workouts to keep things fresh and enjoyable. This approach helps prevent boredom and keeps you engaged in your fitness journey.

## 7. Stay Connected to Your "Why"

Remembering why you started your fitness journey can help you stay motivated through life changes. Whether it's improving your health, boosting your energy levels, or setting a good example for your family, staying connected to your core reasons for pursuing fitness can drive you to maintain your routine.

By implementing these strategies, you can create a sustainable fitness plan that adapts to life's changes while supporting your long-term health and wellness. Consistency, adaptability, and a positive mindset are key components in maintaining a successful fitness journey over time.

## Conclusion

As we reach the end of this journey through fitness, health, and wellness, it's important to reflect on the central message of this book: **fitness is not a one-size-fits-all approach**. Whether you're a beginner starting your first workout, a seasoned athlete, or someone in between, fitness is deeply personal. The key to success lies in understanding your body, your goals, and finding what works for you.

Throughout this book, we have explored various aspects of fitness, from different forms of exercise like **Zumba, Yoga, and Kickboxing**, to the importance of **strength training** and **cardio balance**. We've looked at how fitness is about more than just **lifting weights** or achieving a certain look. True fitness is about **functionality**, **mobility**, and, most importantly, **longevity**.

# The Holistic Approach to Fitness

A central theme we've emphasized is the **holistic nature** of fitness. It's not just about working out in the gym or running miles; it's about integrating **nutrition, recovery, sleep, and mental well-being** into your routine. **Nutrition** plays an essential role in fueling your body, whether your goals are fat loss, muscle gain, or simply maintaining a healthy lifestyle. From understanding **macronutrients** to navigating through the maze of **nutrition myths**, we hope you've gained clarity on how food can be your ally.

We also explored the **science behind recovery**, how crucial it is for muscle growth, injury prevention, and overall performance. It's easy to focus solely on the workouts and forget that the time spent recovering is just as important. Whether it's **hydration**, **stretching**, or simply taking a rest day, recovery is where the magic happens.

# The Role of Motivation and Consistency

Fitness isn't just physical; it requires **mental resilience**. We've touched on the importance of building a **support system**, whether through friends, family, or professional coaching, to help keep you on track. It's in those moments when motivation runs low that having a **coach**, or even engaging with **online fitness communities**, can make all the difference.

And this leads us to one of the most crucial aspects of fitness: **consistency**. The secret to long-term success isn't found in a miracle diet or workout plan but in the **sustainable habits** you form along the way. Whether it's choosing the right foods, scheduling regular workouts, or maintaining proper sleep, fitness is a lifelong commitment to yourself. As we've seen in the section on **setting realistic goals**, achieving fitness isn't about quick fixes—it's about creating a lifestyle that you can maintain over time.

# Fitness for Life

As your body changes through different **life stages**, so too should your fitness approach. What works in your 20s might not be the same in your 40s, but the commitment to maintaining an active, healthy lifestyle should remain. From youth to old age, there's always a way to stay fit, and this book has outlined the tools, techniques, and strategies to do just that.

# Final Thoughts

Remember, fitness is a journey, not a destination. There will be ups and downs, moments of triumph, and times when things don't go as planned. But with the right knowledge, tools, and mindset, you're equipped to take on whatever challenges come your way.

Whether your goal is to run faster, lift heavier, or simply feel better, you now have a roadmap. The journey will always be evolving, but the principles you've learned will serve as a foundation for the rest of your life. You have everything you need to succeed—**the knowledge, the strategies, and the inspiration.**

Now, it's up to you. Take the next step, embrace the process, and continue to grow stronger—both in body and mind. This is your fitness journey, and you're in control.